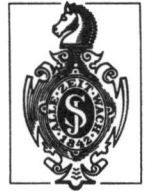

François Lemaire (Ed.)

Mechanical Ventilation

With 58 Figures

Springer-Verlag
Berlin Heidelberg NewYork
London Paris Tokyo
Hong Kong Barcelona Budapest

Professeur Dr. François Lemaire

Medical Director
Service de Réanimation Médicale
Hôpital Henri Mondor
94010 Créteil Cedex, France

Translation of "La ventilation artificielle", 2nd edition
(© Masson, Editeur, Paris, 1991).

ISBN 978-3-540-53322-1   ISBN 978-3-642-87448-2 (eBook)
DOI 10.1007/978-3-642-87448-2

Library of Congress Cataloging-in-Publication Data
Ventilation artificielle. English: Mechanical ventilation/François Lemaire (ed.) p.   cm.
Translation of: La ventilation artificielle. ISBN 978-3-540-53322-1
                                    1. Artificial respiration. 2. Intermittant
positive pressure breathing. 3. High-frequency ventilation. I. Lemaire, François. II. Title.
RC87.9.V4613   1991   617.1′8—dc20   91-162

19/3020-543210— Printed on acid-free paper

Foreword

Only very few therapeutic modalities are used as extensively as mechanical ventilation in intensive care units, during anaesthesia and in emergency situations. Hence theoretical and practical knowledge in this technique had to be made available to workers in a number of medical specialities. In addition to anaesthetists, who are most familiar with artificial ventilation for historical and practical reasons, surgeons, internists, paediatricians and emergency physicians also need a foundation. Furthermore, the widespread application of this life-supporting method requires that paramedical personnel such as nurses and respiratory therapists be trained to use mechanical ventilation, to understand how it works and to be aware of specific side effects and dangers.

This book, edited by François Lemaire, is a well-designed presentation of a number of the relevant aspects, types and problems of mechanical ventilation which are important for physicians and paramedical personnel who use it.

After a description of the technical principles and maintenance of an artificial ventilator, the main part of the book is devoted to the most frequently used types of mechanical respiratory support, with their specific indications, the pathophysiology of their effects on pulmonary gas exchange and the specific choice and regulation of the mechanical variables involved. Older and new types of ventilatory support are discussed; there is a good balance of enough specific information for the inexperienced as well as a critical analysis of the indications for more exotic techniques, such as mandatory minute ventilation, independent lung ventilation and airway pressure release.

Mechanical ventilation during anaesthesia in general and for thoracic surgery in particular are discussed separately. Even if the general principles do not seem very different from those applying to the patient in the intensive care unit, the specific situation merits a specific presentation of ventilation in the operating room.

Two important topics are monitoring and weaning from mechanical ventilation. All too frequently, these points are neglected in daily practice, and important information is lost which could allow a more precise diagnostic and prognostic evaluation. Inappropriate weaning can lead to either unnecessary prolongation of intubation, with the potential danger of pulmonary superinfection and more damage to larynx and trachea, or cardiopulmonary impairment by premature extubation, when cardiovascular adaptation and recovery of respiratory muscle strength are not complete.

Prolonged mechanical ventilation was conceived and introduced in Europe more than 40 years ago and the practice spread to other continents very rapidly. The beginning of the 1990s is certainly an appropriate time to publish a European book on the state of the art of this treatment, one which has saved the lives of so many children and adults during the past decades.

P. M. Suter, Geneva

Acknowledgements. We are grateful to J. L. Meakins and D. Browne for language editing.

List of Contributors

J. B. Andersen
Intensive Care Unit 2042, Rigshospitalet, State Hospital,
Copenhagen University, 2100 Copenhagen ϕ, Denmark

E. Basilico
Istituto di Anestesiologia e Rianimazione,
Universit degli Studi di Milano,
Via F. Sforza, 35, 20122 Milano, Italy

M. Ben Ayed
Department of Intensive Care,
Hôpital Henri Mondor and Medical Bio-Engineering Department,
Paris XII University, 94010 Créteil, France

S. Benito
Servei de Medicina Intensiva, Hospital de la Santa Creu i Sant Pau,
Avda. Sant Antoni Maria Claret, 167, 08025 Barcelona, Spain

O. Boico
Service d'Anesthésie Réanimation, Hôpital Henri Mondor,
94010 Créteil, France

F. Bonnet
Service d'Anesthésie Réanimation, Hôpital Henri Mondor,
94010 Créteil, France

M. Borelli
Istituto di Anestesiologia e Rianimazione,
Universit degli Studi di Milano, Via F. Sforza, 35, 20122 Milano, Italy

A. Braschi
Servizio di Anestesia e Rianimazione l'Settore,
Policlinico S. Matteo I.R.C.C.S., 27100 Pavia, Italy

L. Brochard
Medical Intensive Care Unit, INSERM U 296 and Paris XII University,
Hôpital Henri Mondor, 94010 Créteil, France

D. R. G. Browne
Department of Anaesthesia, Royal Free Hospital, London NW3 2O6, U.K.

C. Brun-Buisson
Service de Réanimatin Médicale, Hôpital Henri Mondor, 94010 Créteil,
France

G. Conti
Institute of Anaesthesiology and Intensive Care, ICU,
University La Sapienza, 00100 Rome, Italy

K. J. Falke
Department of Anaesthesiology, Klinikum R. Virchow, Free University,
1000 Berlin 65, F.R.G.

M.-J. Fevrier
Service d'Anesthésie Réanimation, Hôpital Henri Mondor,
94010 Créteil, France

M. Fischler
Départment d'Anesthésie Réanimation, Hôpital Foch, 92151 Suresnes,
France

L. Gattinoni
Istituto di Anestesiologia e Rianimazione,
Universit degli Studi di Milano, Via F. Sforza, 35, 20122 Milano, Italy

G. Iotti
Servizio di Anestesia e Rianimazione l'Settore,
Policlinico S. Matteo I.R.C.C.S., 27100 Pavia, Italy

J.-P. Laaban
Department of Pneumology and Intensive Care,
75004 Hôtel-Dieu de Paris, France

F. Lemaire
Service de Réanimation Médicale, Hôpital Henri Mondor, 94010 Créteil,
France

J. Marty
Départment d'Anesthésie et de Réanimation Chirurgicale, Hôpital Bichat,
46, Rue Henri-Huchard, 75018 Paris, France

D. Mascheroni
Istituto die Anestesiologia e Rianimazione,
Universit degli Studi di Milano, Via F. Sforza, 35, 20122 Milano, Italy

J. L. Meakins
Department of Surgery and ICU, Royal Victoria Hospital,
Magill University, Montreal H3A 1A1, Canada

Y. Nivoche
Départment d'Anesthésie et de Réanimation Chirurgicale, Hôpital Bichat,
46, Rue Henri-Huchard, 75018 Paris, France

A. Pesenti
Istituto di Anestesiologia e Rianimazione,
Universit degli Studi di Milano, Via F. Sforza, 35, 20122 Milano, Italy

A. Pilorget
Department of Anesthesiology and Intensive Care II,
Hôpital Henri Mondor, 94010 Créteil, France

J. Räsänen
Department of Anesthesiology, Childrens's Hospital,
University of Helsinki, 00290 Helsinki, Finland

P. Rieuf
Intensive Care Unit, Hôpital Henri Mondor, 94010 Créteil, France

P. Tassin
Intensive Care Unit, Hôpital Henri Mondor, 94010 Créteil, France

F. Trémolières
Service de Médecine Interne, Centre Hospitalier Fanis Quesnay,
78201 Mantes la Jolie, France

Contents

XII   Contents

Mechanical Ventilation

Description of a Ventilator

F. Trémolières

Artificial ventilation, first brought into clinical use more than 30 years ago, is now a standard form of therapy. Its increased efficacy owes as much to technological advances as to the improving skill of physicians. However, a ventilator cannot be operated as easily as, say, a washing machine. Its application requires both a knowledge of state-of-the art medical science and a thorough understanding of the equipment and how it functions. Also, it must be stressed that while the principles regarding how a ventilator operates are simple, there are now very sophisticated machines available which can adapt to almost any clinical situation.

Over the past 35 years 300–400 different types of ventilators have been marketed, and this variety attests to the difficulties encountered in designing the ideal ventilator. The clinically useful ventilator only results from a compromise between conflicting needs.

A short section will be devoted here to a description of the different types of ventilators and to the practical problems arising in selecting the right equipment. However, there will be no discussion concerning the specific ventilators currently available since their rapid obsolescence would invalidate any such list. This technological approach to ventilators will be completed by a description of the most common features [inspiratory flow, pause, inspiratory/expiratory (I/E) ratio] and of the ventilatory modes (controlled mechanical ventilation (CMV), synchronized intermittent mandatory ventilation (SIMV), positive end expiratory pressure (PEEP), or continuous positive airway pressure (CPAP).

Physical Properties of Ventilators

Insufflation Phase

Artificial ventilation achieves a periodic transfer of gases between two mechanical systems: the ventilator and the thorax-lung. Accordingly, a ventilator always includes a gas source which delivers a preset volume of gas into the patient. This gas source is the driving force and the energy is provided either by a compressed gas cylinder or by a mechanical system compressing room air (see Fig. 1 for a diagram of the mechanical characteristics of a ventilator) (Peslin 1969).

Whatever operating principle the ventilator relies upon, it may be represented as a pressure source (Ps) developing an internal resistance (Ri), and

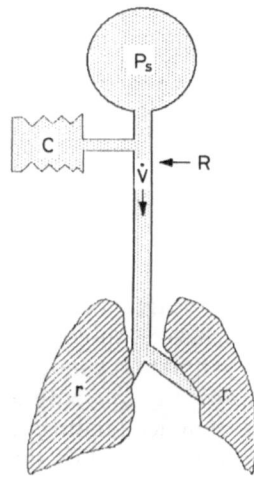

Fig. 1. Schematic diagram of a ventilator. P_s, pressure source; R, internal resistance; C, total compliance; V, instantaneous flow; r, airways resistance

connected to the patient via a compressible system (circuit) with a compliance (Ci). The thorax-lung system's compliance (Cp) opposes a resistance (Rp) to the transfer of the gas which is represented by the instantaneous flow ($\dot{V}$).

Alveolar pressure (P_A) is a function of both the flow and the total resistance (R). The total resistance is the sum of the ventilator's internal resistance and of the airway resistance: $R = Ri + Rp$.

The equation is the following:

$$\dot{V} = (Ps - P_A)/R \tag{1}$$

where $\dot{V}$ is expressed in l/s, P in cm H_2O, and R in cm H_2O/l/s.

In addition, the insufflated volume may be calculated at any time provided compliance is known.

To simplify the equation, we shall asume that the ventilator compliance is zero or, at least, very small and assimilate the patient's compliance (Cp) into total compliance (C).

$$\dot{V} = P_A \times C. \tag{2}$$

The graphic representation of Eq. (1) (Fig. 2) is referred to as the "flow-pressure relationship". If Ps is constant, the curve is linear; its slope is

$$\Delta P/\Delta V = -1/R.$$

This equation means that a ventilator with a high internal resistance (slope close to zero) will provide flows which depend only slightly, if at all, on the insufflation pressure, i.e., on the mechanical characteristics of the patient. On the other hand, a ventilator with a low internal resistance is not expected to maintain a constant ventilatory flow should the mechanical characteristics of the patient worsen.

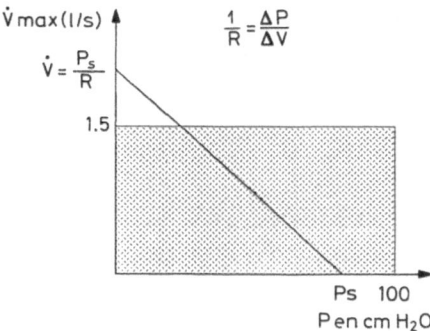

Fig. 2. Flow pressure relationship (when outside the gray area, a ventilator becomes a volume generator)

There are basically, two types of ventilators:

1. Those with a low driving pressure—entailing low internal resistance—whose performance is influenced by the downstream conditions (known as pressure ventilators).
2. Those with a high driving pressure—a high internal resistance—whose performance is not much influenced by downstream conditions (known as volume generators).

In fact, there are not two different types of ventilators but only one; indeed, it is the value of the driving pressure which characterizes the two ways in which the ventilator may operate.

In the first ventilators, the driving pressure generally changed during the insufflation depending on the mechanical characteristics of the motor assembly (pump, plunger, bellows). Thus, the instantaneous flow varied during the inspiratory phase while tidal volume remained constant; these ventilators were known as *volume generators*. The way flow would change during insufflation was a specific feature of each ventilator. In most cases, the flow pattern was grossly a sine wave; flow first increased to a peak value and then decreased until the end of the insufflation. This was the flow pattern of the early Engström ventilators (150 and 300). The way flow varied would eventually be modified through the setting of the machine's "insufflation rate" control.

Recently manufactured ventilators allow the selection of more precise flow patterns during the inspiratory phase, thus providing continuous, accelerating, decelerating, or sine wave flows (Pulmosystem Z800, Draeger Eva, Kontron 4100S, Veolar, Bennet 5000). This regulation is achieved through the electronic control of pressure changes, or, if the driving pressure of the ventilator remains constant, through the modification of the internal resistance of the machine. A programmed variation of the pressure may be obtained using a step motor (Kontron 4100) or a microprocessor-controlled servovalve (Engström Erica).

Modifying the internal resistance of the ventilator is a frequent mode of ventilation in advanced servoregulated ventilators, such as the Servo-Ventilator 900. In this equipment, the minute variation of the ventilator's internal resistance, controlled by an electrovalve, determines the characteristics of the instantaneous flow. For example, in order to maintain a constant flow with a low working pressure (40 cm H_2O) and to insufflate a volume of 0.5 l in 1 s, when the alveolar pressure reaches 30 cm H_2O at the end of the inspiration, resistance should vary as follows:

constant $\dot V = 0.5$ l/s,

Ri at a time $0 = (Ps-Pa)/V = (40-0)/0.5 = 80$ cm H_2O/l/s,

Ri at the end of insufflation $= (40-30)/0.5 = 20$ cm H_2O/l/s.

At present, advances in electronics permit the design of ventilators which are low pressure generators that may become volume generators; i.e., the parameters delivered are unaffected by the mechanical changes occurring at the patient level. This is possible because the instantaneous changes in the driving pressure or in the internal resistance of the ventilator may be monitored.

With respect to classical design, the present section reminds us that

1. Only those ventilators whose instantaneous flow cannot be markedly influenced by mechanical changes occurring in the patient's thorax-lung system are suitable for prolonged artificial ventilation.
2. Only financial consideration (pressure ventilators are generally simpler and less expensive) or specific clinical indications may lead to the selection of a pressure ventilator.

However, such a strict attitude may be tempered. Present monitoring devices, especially with regard to measurement and the continuous display of the expired instantaneous flow, allow the use of a ventilator even though it lacks in efficiency (with respect to the accepted criteria), provided it is capable of actually indicating at any time the true ventilation of the patient.

Expiratory Phase

The theoretical approach to the expiratory phase is a complement of the above. The source pressure is now the atmospheric pressure which is assumed to be the baseline pressure. During this phase, the ventilator generally operates in a passive way. It may only act through resistance to gas flow opposed by the expiratory arm of the circuit. Sometimes, a resistance may be willingly set up to maintain a positive end expiratory pressure (PEEP) greater than atmospheric pressure.

Cycling Mode

The cycling mode determines the parameter(s) which control(s) the switching from inspiratory phase to expiratory phase and vice-versa. Five mechanisms may control artificial ventilation cycling:

1. Time: Switching from one phase to another or passing from one cycle to the next is automatically initiated at the end of a preset time interval.

2. Volume: Switching from one phase to the next occurs when a preset volume has been insufflated or expired.
3. Pressure: The next phase occurs when the pressure within airways reaches a preset level.
4. Flow: Cycling is initiated by the decrease of volume down to a preset value.
5. Patient: Switching from one phase to the next occurs when the patient attempts to inspire.

The first four mechanisms may act as signals for either expiration or insufflation while the fifth may only determine the switching from expiration to insufflation.

Practically, in advanced ventilators, the switching from expiration to insufflation is usually time-controlled; this ensures a fixed frequency of cycles. However, the triggering of the insufflation by the patient himself is a technique often used in conventional artificial ventilation: it is the present "assist-controlled ventilation" (assist-CMV), as opposed to the exclusively "controlled mechanical ventilation" (CMV). It often results in an increasing frequency of respiratory cycles at the expense of the expiratory phase, while the duration and the volume of the insufflation remain unchanged (sometimes, tidal volume is increased). In all cases, the minute-volume is increased proportionally to the frequency.

This triggering mechanism is most important in the ventilatory modes using the patient's inspiratory efforts, in which the synchronization of controlled cycles with the patient is a main feature for his well-being and even more for the efficacy of the method—continuous mechanical ventilation (CMV, SIMV, MMV, spontaneous, pressure support—see Sects. 3, 4, 5 and 6).

Things are somewhat more complex when switching from inspiration to expiration. Table 1, taking into account the motor characteristics of the ventilator, shows that flow-controlled cycling is almost never used. It may be seen that these ventilators which are time-cycled high pressure generators (or the equivalent such as the Servo 900), have inspiratory characteristics completely unaffected by what may occur at the patient level. In the same group, ventilators

Table 1. Control of instantaneous flow, insufflation time, and tidal volume according to the different configurations of ventilators

	Cycling mode	$\dot{V}_i$	T_i	V_T
High pressure generator or equivalent	Time	+	+	+
	Volume	+	−	+
	Pressure	+	−	−
Low pressure generator	Time	−	+	−
	Volume	−	−	+
	Pressure	−	−	−

The sign + indicates that the variable is controlled by the ventilator only; the sign − indicates that the variable is controlled by both the ventilator and the patient.

whose cycling mode depends on the volume are almost identical to those of the previous group. However, although flow is assumed to be constant, a 10% decrease is frequently seen when the downstream resistance rises very much. For example, this may occur on the Bourns Bear I which, under drastic conditions, maintains a constant tidal volume, at the cost of a slight increase in insufflation time. Frequency is not modified; I/T ratio (the inspiratory phase as a percent of the total respiratory cycle) increases.

An intermediate situation exists in certain ventilators where switching from the inspiratory to the expiratory phase is time-controlled. However, inspiration actually includes two phases: an active period which is the true insufflation time, volume-cycled, whose duration varies as a function of flow; and a passive time when insufflation has ended, but expiration has not yet started. During this period, flow is zero, the intrapulmonary volume remains constant, and alveolar pressure stabilizes more or less rapidly to the thorax relaxation pressure level for a given volume. This pressure is a function of the thorax-lung static compliance which can be evaluated. This latter phase is the "pause" at the end of the insufflation, also known as a "plateau." This feature exists in Engström ventilators.

In all the other ventilators, two or three parameters depend on the patient and there is no means to predict, prior to connecting the patient, how efficient the ventilation will be and whether or not it will change with time.

Basic Features

The diagram presented in Fig. 3 applies to all ventilators; it provides a simple picture that users should always bear in mind.

A ventilator may be represented as a source of gas (G) which is the driving system. Its energy comes from either a compressed gas bottle feeding the ventilator or a mechanical system compressing a gas mixture drawn at the atmospheric pressure. The gas source is connected to the patient by the

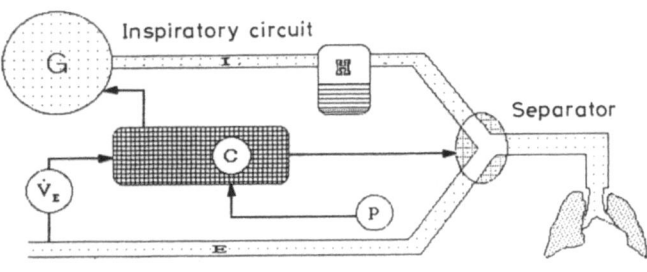

Fig. 3. Description of a ventilator. *G*, gas source; *I*, inspiratory branch) *E*, expiratory branch; *S*, separator; *H*, humidifier; *P*, pressure manometer; *V*, flowmeter measuring the instantaneous expired flow; *C*, control systems

inspiratory tubing (I) through which the gas mixture flows during insufflation. Expired gas is discharged through the expiratory tubing (E). Circuits E and I are separated at the end of a common piece which allows connection of the ventilator to the patient's intubation canula or tracheostomy tube. A system of valves, forming the circuit separator (S), prevents inspiratory gas from flowing into the expiratory branch during insufflation and the expired gas from entering the inspiratory arm during expiration (rebreathing). This circuit separator is either placed at the beginning of the common piece, as on the diagram, or inside the ventilator itself. Regardless of its position in the circuit, any system occluding the expiratory side of the respiratory circuit while opening the inspiratory branch during insufflation and vice-versa during expiration is capable of operating as a separator.

The control system (C) of the mechanical part is an essential element of the ventilator. It sets the characteristics of the respiratory cycle: insufflation time, expiration time, duration of an inspiratory pause, % cycle times, volume of insufflated gas, minute flow, and mode of ventilation. It initiates the respiratory cycle and synchronizes the operation of the separator's valves (either electronic, mechanical, or pneumatic).

The quality and performance of the ventilator depend on both the mechanical characteristics of the pressure source and the control system.

In addition to these basic elements, a ventilator includes essential accessories: a system to humidify the insufflated gases saturated with water vapor at a temperature neighboring 30 °C (H) and a system to monitor artificial ventilation, measuring:

1. The pressure (manometer P). This pressure is usually measured at a site within the ventilator, distant from the patient. In most cases this distance is not a drawback (especially in adults). However, in some instances, it may be important to measure the intratracheal pressure, especially when the resistance opposed to gas flow is high, i.e., in small-sized intubation tubes.
2. The expiratory instantaneous flow (flowmeter V_E). This measurement is considered essential for the monitoring and safety of the patient in advanced monitors, even in ventilators that are to be used over short periods of time (in the operating room, especially).

Setting Parameters for Artificial Ventilation

Setting the artificial ventilation parameters is an important task for the operator. It includes an initial or "a priori" setting time prior to connecting the patient. Checking the effects of the initial setting leads to further adjustments and assumes that the operator:

1. Has a precise idea of the physical properties and keeps the diagram of a ventilator in mind.
2. Is thoroughly familiar with the particular ventilator being used.

3. Has personally checked the ventilator for adequate setting and correct operation.

Basic Parameters

The basic parameters of artificial ventilation are:

1. Tidal volume (V_T).
2. Frequency (F).
3. Inspired minute volume (V_I).

Setting two of these parameters determines the third one. The frequency determines the duration of the respiratory cycle (period). Thus, the easiest way to set the parameters consists in setting either the frequency and the tidal volume or the frequency and the inspiratory flow.

In addition to these parameters many ventilators require a setting for peak flow during insufflation (Bear I, Engström Erica, Pneumotron 80). This changes neither the tidal volume, nor the frequency, nor of course the insufflated minute volume, but it determines the I/E ratio (Bear I) or the occurrence of an inspiratory hold (Engström Erica).

The above basic parameters may also be selected indirectly by setting the value for peak flow, whether it should remain constant or not during insufflation, and simultaneously both the insufflation and the expiration times, insufflation, and simultaneously both the insufflation and the expiration times, or either of these parameters and the I/E ratio. This setting, unusual in France, is rather common in Anglo-Saxon countries (Oxford Ventilator, and partially Monaghan, Ohio). In the absence of specific indicators, this mode of control is not easy to use. It entails a trial-and-error method before a proper setting is obtained. Indeed, the frequency may be known only after various calculations; and the tidal volume, or the flow, is only known after the patient is connected.

The CPU 1 Ohmeda is arranged in that fashion; however, it is simple to use and reliable. Indeed, the setting is precise. One control sets flow (liters per minute) in the range 0–120 l/min, i.e., 0–2 l/s. Three controls set the insufflation time, pause, and expiration time. Simultaneously, the computer of the ventilator displays the values for frequency, insufflated tidal volume, inspiratory flow, and I/E ratio, which are fully determined by the setting of the parameters described above. This technique, though it may seem more complex than the usual methods, sets any characteristic of the respiratory cycle, using four controls, not only for controlled ventilation, but also for those ventilation modes which combine ventilator-controlled cycles with spontaneous breathing (CMV, SIMV, MMV). This ventilator has a simpler control board than the front panel of other machines using more conventional basic settings but necessitating extra controls to determine the CMV, SIMV, and MMV (Bear I and II, Servo 900C, Bennet 5000, Veolar Hamilton, Draëger Eva, Engström Erica). Adapting the setting mode of the CPU 1 is quite achievable. However, this type of setting requires some minimal efforts from the whole team so that any member may set up the ventilator correctly.

O_2 Concentration

The F_{1O_2} is almost always selected directly using the air/oxygen mixer scale ranging from 0.21 to 1 (21%–100% oxygen). The precision and especially the stability of most mixers is generally quite sufficient for clinical use, provided gas source pressures do not vary too widely. These mixers require both air and oxygen sources, compressed to 2–3 bars or more.

Other Settings—Ventilation Modes

The other settings concern the different characteristics of the respiratory cycle (sigh, plateau, I/T ratio, inspiratory flow pattern, PEEP, inspiratory pressure support), and the different modes of ventilation (CV, assit-CMV, IMV-SIMV, MMV, PEEP-CPAP). Although most of these have long been described, they became operational only recently owing to advances in electronics and microprocessor technologies. Among these settings, the most important are fully detailed elsewhere in the text (PEEP, SIMV, CPAP, inspiratory pressure support, MMV).

The following paragraphs will describe the "sigh," I/E ratio, pause, and assisted-controlled modes of ventilation.

A *sigh* is a periodic hyperinflation. This feature allows to deliver, at preset intervals, one or several cycles with increased tidal volumes. Its indication seems rather reduced at present if a sufficient insufflated volume has been set, and especially if a low level of PEEP is used (3–5 cm H_2), maintaining a sufficient functional residual capacity (FRC).

The *I/T ratio* defines the duration of the inspiratory phase as a percent of total respiratory cycle (T = period). This ratio is better than the conventional I/E ratio (inspiration/expiration). Standard I/T ratios range from 0.25 to 0.50 where insufflation represents 25%–50% of the whole cycle and corresponds to an I/E ratio range of 1/3 to 1/1. An I/T ratio greater than 0.50 (50%) is sometimes useful (Baker et al. 1982a, b; Boros 1979; Mannino et al. 1976; Spahr et al. 1980; Stewart et al. 1981).

An *inspiratory hold* known as a *plateau* (or *pause*) may be managed during the zero flow period at the end of the insufflation. The inspiratory time includes two phases; the first is active, the second is passive (inspiratory hold). Using a plateau to optimize the alveolar ventilation may seem of no obvious clinical value. However, provided it is long enough (0.5–1 s), it may help determine the pressure at the end of the pause. This pressure may be used to evaluate the mechanical characteristics of the ventilator while the patient cannot interfere.

Figure 4 summarizes the different flow patterns theoretically available:

1. "Square" or "continuous" flow pattern: flow reaches at first shot its peak value and remains constant throughout the insufflation time.

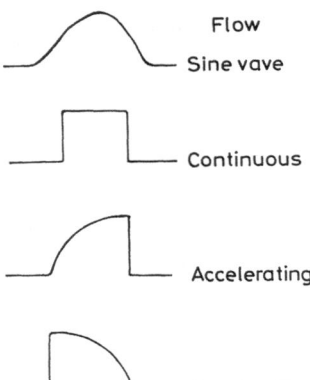

Fig. 4. Variation of instantaneous flow during insufflation

2. "Accelerating" flow pattern: flow increases progressively to a maximum value at the end of insufflation.
3. "Decelerating" flow pattern: flow decreases progressively from a peak value to zero at the end of insufflation.
4. "Sine wave" flow pattern: the last curve of the figure simply illustrates any other pattern possibly evoking a "sine wave" variation of flow whose characteristics are adjustable in some advanced sophisticated ventilators.

Practically, if the ventilator in use allows such settings, which pattern should be selected and which criteria are important?

The literature on artificial ventilation includes many studies emphasizing the advantages of one or another insufflation mode (Baker et al. 1982a, b; Boros 1979; Dammann et al. 1978; Jansson and Jonson 1972). Actually, no spectacular information comes to light from any of these studies.

It should be kept in mind that:

1. Evidence is lacking in support of using sine wave flow patterns.
2. When similar tidal volumes are being insufflated, peak insufflation pressure never reaches as high a level as obtained with either a continuous or a decelerating flow. To simplify and facilitate calculations during recording of ventilatory data, a continuous flow is best. Using a decelerating flow has been recommended together with prolonged insufflation times (Mannino et al. 1976); however, this usually generates a smaller insufflated minute volume than preset. Thus, in this situation, flow should be monitored with the expiratory flowmeter.

Controlled Ventilation vs Assist-Controlled Ventilation

Definitions

Controlled Mechanical Ventilation. Mechanical ventilation in which the respiratory cycle is completely determined by the setting of the ventilator controls and is unaffected by the patient is called controlled mechanical ventilation (CMV). Controlled respiratory cycle indicates a mechanical respiratory cycle the parameters of which depend on the ventilator control settings.

Assist-Controlled Mechanical Ventilation. Mechanical ventilation in which the patient may trigger the insufflation of a preset tidal volume at a frequency that he determines is known as assist-controlled mechanical ventilation (assist-CMV). A minimum back-up frequency is ensured by the ventilator. Assisted cycle indicates a mechanical respiratory cycle whose insufflation is triggered by the patient.

Controlled Mechanical Ventilation

Figure 5 shows the pressure and flow profiles during controlled mechanical respiratory cycles. To be perfectly efficient, controlled ventilation where the patient cannot modify the cycle characteristics entails either an absence of spontaneous movements of the patient or his perfect, spontaneous or drug-induced, adaptation to the ventilator.

Assist-Controlled Mechanical Ventilation

In this ventilation mode, the patient initiates a respiratory cycle whose characteristics depend on the a priori settings of the ventilator. The importance of this mode is generally underrated; however, to evaluate a given ventilator, it is essential to be aware that the ventilators available at present offer two different assist-CMV.

Type 1. T he Servo type is the assist-CMV available in the Servo 900. As shown in Fig. 6, any inspiratory effort of the patient, provided it reaches a preset sensitivity threshold, triggers, whenever this effort occurs, the insufflation of an assisted cycle. In practice, these inspiratory efforts will increase the cycle frequency and, proportionally, the minute ventilation. The increase in the ventilation frequency is only limited by the technical possibilities of the ventilator used and the necessity of maintaining an adequate expiration time.

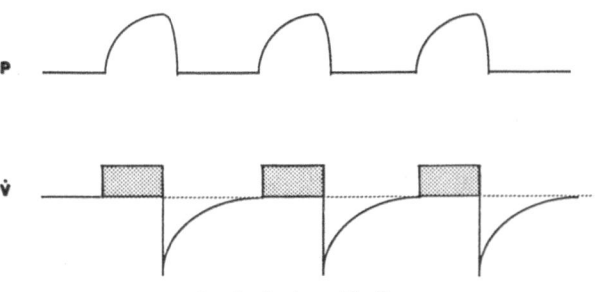

P

V̇

Controlled ventilation

Fig. 5. Controlled ventilation: pressure-flow

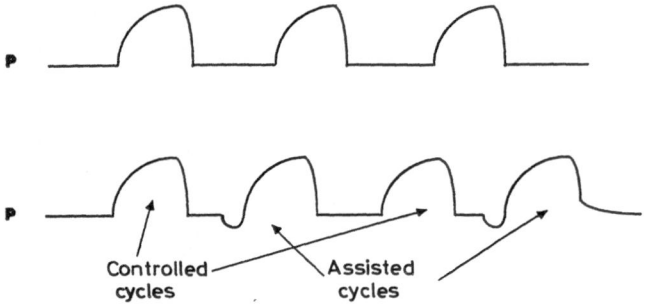

Controlled cycles — Assisted cycles

Fig. 6. Assist-CMV, type I (Servo)

To illustrate this mode, we shall study a practical case. A ventilator is set as follows: frequency, 20; tidal volume (V_t), 1 l; I/E ratio, 1/2 (i.e., I/T, 0.33) providing an insufflation time of 1 s. Assuming that the patient experiences polypnea and attempts to inspire 30 times per min, then the respiratory (patient-triggered) frequency changes to 30/min; V_t remains unchanged (1 l); the I/E ratio becomes 1/1 (i.e., I/T = 0.5), and the minute ventilation reaches 30 l.

In a tachypneic and hypoxic patient, ill-adapted to the ventilator (a condition which worsens his respiratory status), the flexibility to synchronize the ventilator cycles with the patient's need allows improvement in the oxygen supply to the patient and, at best, his adaptation to the preset frequency. This mode is a good means for difficult patients and, because it is safe, should be attempted prior to using any other technique.

This ventilation mode will be effective, provided:

1. The response time of the system (i.e., the lag time between the beginning of the patient's inspiratory effort and the onset of the mechanical insufflation) is as short as possible; in practice, this delay should be less than 200 ms.
2. The ventilator includes an operator-adjustable triggering level, not so much to compel the patient to make a great effort to initiate a mandatory cycle, but to prevent the occurrence of an excessively high triggering frequency, should the patient's effort be too small.

To optimize this mode of ventilation, the operator should measure the patient's spontaneous frequency and set the respirator frequency just below it. In tachypneic patients (frequency > 50), it may be useful to set the ventilator frequency to one-half the spontaneous frequency. We are unaware of a study suggesting that this mode of ventilation, particularly in hypoxemic and ill-adapted patients, is better than controlled ventilation. However, common sense and experience teach us that when correctly used, this technique allows to adapt more patients using fewer sedative drugs. When the Servo 900 was marketed, the practitioners, once they had become familiar with the machine, recognized its superiority over the other ventilators available at that time. Indeed, some had an

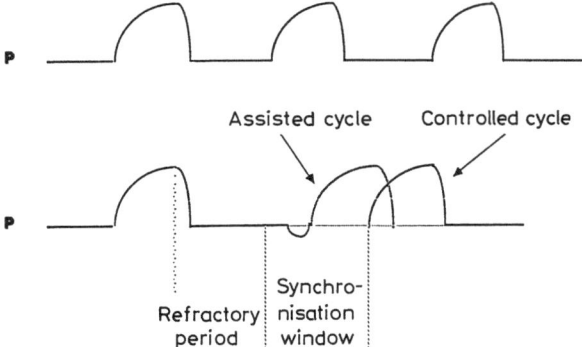

Fig. 7. Assist-CMV, type II

assist-CMV feature, but its characteristics (especially an excessively long response time) did not allow a correct use of this mode.

Type 2. The second type of assist-controlled ventilations is very different from the first. The cycling in this mode is illustrated by Fig. 7. At the end of a normal mandatory insufflation, there is a "refractory" phase during which no assisted respiratory cycle may be triggered by the patient, as in controlled ventilation. At the end of this period, which usually corresponds to the normal duration of the expiration as fixed by the a priori settings, a "window" (or synchronization time) starts. During that period of time, a cycle may occur only in response to the patient's inspiratory effort. If there is no demand from the patient at the end of this synchronization time, the ventilator initiates a controlled cycle. Thus, this mode always leads to a reduction of frequency. However, in case the patient fails to trigger respiratory cycles, a back-up frequency is ensured by the ventilator. It depends on the duration of the refractory period and on the synchronization window, and ranges approximately between 10 and 12 insufflations per minute, in most ventilators.

The aim of this second type of assist-controlled ventilation is much different to that of the Servo type described above. It has long been used as a weaning technique to promote the reeducation of the patient, since it is the effort required to trigger a mandatory cycle which is progressively increased.

At present, the first type of assist-CMV is useful for many indications, while the second type is by far supplanted by more recent modes using a combination of controlled (or assisted) cycles with spontaneous breaths, such as the SIMV, MMV, or inspiratory support (see the following section). The ventilators including the first type of assist-CMV (Servo) may sometimes be used during the weaning period; however, the reverse is impossible.

To conclude, using the CV mode is justified when the patient has no spontaneous activity (anesthesia, coma) or when he is perfectly well adapted to the machine. On the other hand, we see no reason for not using the assist-controlled mode extensively.

Barometric Modes

These modes were available on a few machines (CPU 1, Omheda); however, they rapidly lost their attractiveness since they were merely the rediscovery of the "pressure relaxation" incorporated into highly sophisticated ventilators (see beginning of section). The insufflated volume is defined by both insufflation flow and peak pressure. These barometric modes were soon changed in "inspiratory support."

Technological Evolution—the Different Types of Ventilators

Practical Indications for the Selection of a Ventilator

It seems difficult to describe the technological evolution of ventilators in detail; every (or almost every) new machine brought—or claimed to bring—its small contribution to the advancement of technology.

We shall indicate only the main steps:

1. In 1952, the Engström ventilator facilitated taking under complete charge any distressed patient, thus ensuring an efficient "controlled ventilation." For more than 15 years this remained the most advanced of the ventilators.
2. In 1956 a purely pneumatic machine was designed in France, the RPR (Rosenstiel, Pesty, Richard). In spite of unspectacular performance, it was the most widely distributed in France (especially in surgical wards) and was produced for nearly 30 years.
3. The pneumatic logical cells allowed (in the early 1960s) the design of very small but very powerful ventilators requiring no compressed gas as fuel source. Their use exclusively as back-up and transport ventilations was confirmed with the years.
4. Electronics facilitated the smashing entry onto the market (in the 1970s) of the Servo 900. With regard to controlled ventilation, this ventilator is not better than the earlier ones. However, the advantages of this new generation compelled rapid recognition: their size was reduced; the settings were precise; they were more reliable and less expensive to maintain; and above all they allowed practical adaptation of the ventilator to the patient's needs.

    Electronics, and now microprocessors, have changed the face of ventilator technology. From this revolution stemmed an evolution of artificial ventilation towards better efficacy and greater safety.

The ventilators designed for prolonged ventilation generally have the most technical features and the newest ventilation modes. Depending on their performance, they will be listed as middle-range or high-tech which will be reflected in the cost. They take up the greatest share of the equipment on the intensive care ward.

There are specific ventilators adapted to very particular situations; home ventilation, equipment for respiratory reeducation, emergency and transport ventilation, ventilation during and after surgery, neonatology.

Practically, selecting an adequate ventilator involves:

1. The determination of actual needs: definition of the type(s) of ventilator(s) required (prolonged ventilation and/or specific techniques).
2. The evaluation of the equipment already on the ward; an important point for the efficiency and cost of maintenance and repairs and for the quality and safety of ventilation managed by a large team.
3. Having balanced these elements, a comparison of the different ventilators requires

   —Performance of a personnel and real-time test of the machine prior to purchase.
   —A second opinion from a qualified colleague experienced with the ventilator.
   —Validation from recent publication (equipment performance).

All of the above may seem of secondary importance when compared with the material in the following chapters. However, we remain convinced that a thorough knowledge, even if it is schematic, of "what is a ventilator," is essential for optimal use of the equipment. The efficacy and the safety of ventilation depend on such sound knowledge.

References

Baker AB, Restall R, Clark BW (1982a) Effects of varying inspiratory flow waveform and time in intermittent positive pressure ventilation: emphysema. Br J Anaesth 54:547–553

Baker AB, Thompson JB, Turner J, Hansen P (1982b) Effects of varying inspiratory flow waveform and time in intermittent positive pressure ventilation: pulmonary oedema. Br J Anaesth 54:539–546

Boros SJ (1979) Variations in inspiratory/expiratory ratio and airway pressure wave form during mechanical ventilation: the significance of mean airway pressure. J Pediatr 94(1):114–117

Cazala JB, Louville J, Weber B, et al. (1984) Respirateurs; fonctions et usages. Agressologie 25 (2,3,4)

Chopin C, et al. (1985) Monitoring de la ventilation. In: Réanimation et médecine d'urgence. Expansion Scientifique, Paris, pp 63–130

Dammann JF, MacAslan TC, Maffeo CJ (1978) Optimal flow pattern for mechanical ventilation of the lungs. II. The effect of a sine versus square wave flow pattern with and without an end-inspiratory pause on patients. Crit Care Med 6(5):293–310

Hayes B (1982) Ventilation and ventilators. J Med Eng Technol 6(5):177–192

Jansson L, Jonson B (1972) A theoretical study on flow patterns of ventilators. Scand J Respir Dis 53:237–246

Lindahl S (1979) Influence of an end inspiratory pause on pulmonary ventilation, gas distribution, and lung perfusion during artificial ventilation. Crit Care Med 7(12):540–546

Mannino FL, Feldman BH, Heldt GP, DeLue NA, Wimmer JE, Fletcher MA, Gluck L (1976) Early mechanical ventilation in RDS with a prolonged inspiration. Pediatr Res 10:464–471

Mushin WW, Rendel Baker L, Thompson PW, Mapleson WW (1980) On automatic ventilation of the lung, 3rd edn. Blackwell, Oxford
Osborn JJ (1978) A flow meter for respiratory monitoring. Crit Care Med 6:349–351
Peslin R (1969) The physical properties of ventilators in the inspiratory phase. Anesthesiology 30:315–324
Spahr RC, Klein AM, Brown DR, MacDonald HM, Holzman IR (1980) Hyaline membrane disease. A controlled study of inspiratory to expiratory ratio in its management by ventilator. Am J Dis Child 134:373–376
Stewart AR, Finer NN, Peters KL (1981) Effects of alternations of inspiratory and expiratory pressures and inspiratory/expiratory ratio on mean airway pressure, blood gases and intractranial pressue. Pedaitr 67(4):474–480
Tremolières F, Morizet-Mahoudeaux P (1981) Les respirateurs. In: Broun G, Moreau C (eds) Les équipments biomédicaux. Maloine, Paris, pp 389–404
Tremolières F, et al. (1983) Choix d'un respirateur. In: Réanimation et médecine d'urgence. Expansion Scintifique, Paris pp 253–334

Positive End Expiratory Pressure

F. Lemaire and C. Brun-Buisson

Positive end expiratory pressure (PEEP) was first used during the 1930s as part of the therapy for pulmonary edema, and later, during World War II, by airplane pilots. However, widespread use of PEEP as a therapeutic method started only after the description of acute respiratory distress syndrome (ARDS) (Ashbaugh et al. 1967). Early studies showed that the improvement of PaO_2 induced by PEEP was related to an increase in lung volume (Falke et al. 1972; Ramachandran and Fairley 1970), corresponding to the fact that the intrapulmonary shunt responsible for hypoxemia in ARDS is determined by alveolar edema and collapse.

However, the deleterious effects of PEEP on hemodynamics (decreased blood pressure and cardiac output) and oxygen transport were reported as early as 1972 (Lutch and Murray 1972; Suter et al. 1975). During the past 20 years, an incredibly high number of publications have facilitated a thorough understanding of the pathophysiological aspects of PEEP. However, it is important to realize that such a universally used technique, and one so well investigated, has never been adequately shown to improve the survival of patients with ARDS.

Technical Aspects

All modern ventilators have some built-in device producing PEEP (Spearman 1988). Spontaneous breathing with PEEP is also possible (with continuous positive airway pressure, CPAP), using the same devices, when the patient breathes through the ventilator tubing or by using any kind of continuous flow system.

All PEEP devices currently used are more or less of the threshold type: expiratory flow is opposed by applying a relatively constant force until flow stops completely and a valve closes abruptly. Many valves, however, exhibit some flow resisting properties, implying that the level of PEEP is not steady, but increases with the expiratory flow (Marini et al. 1985; Pinsky et al. 1988). Most PEEP systems are spring-loaded devices and exhalation valve balloons, as underwater columns and water weighted diaphragms are now rarely used. Some ventilators use electro-mechanical valves to control expiratory flow. The Hamilton Veolar uses an electromagnetic pin which controls a diaphragm placed at the expiratory port. The Siemens Servo 900C uses a scissor-valve which modulates the expiratory flow and can create PEEP. All these devices are relatively accurate and provide a reliable level of PEEP; all augment the expiratory resistance and increase the expiratory work of breathing when patients breathe spontaneously.

Pulmonary Mechanics

A reduction of functional residual capacity (FRC) is a major characteristic of ARDS (Table 1), and the main function of PEEP is to restore FRC towards normal values (Fig. 1). When applied in five patients with ARDS, MacIntyre et al. (1969) measured an increase of FRC by 30% ± 13% (500 ml) by applying 5 cm H_2O PEEP. Similarly, Kumar et al. (1970) found FRC was increased by an average 1.21, when using 13 cm H_2O PEEP. Augmentation of lung volume with PEEP is not obtained instantaneously: it takes five breaths after application of PEEP to reach 90% of the entire variation (Katz 1981).

Falke et al. (1972) demonstrated that compliance was increased when PEEP was applied to ARDS patients. Suter et al. (1975), in a now classical article coined the term "best PEEP" to identify the level of PEEP beyond which compliance began to decrease, due to alveolar distension. This biphasic pattern of compliance when PEEP is increased stepwise, is explained by the curvilinear shape of the pulmonary pressure volume (P–V) curve. Matamis et al. (1984) using a 2-l syringe, traced such P–V curves in patients with ARDS; in recent-onset ARDS, associated with florid edema, they documented such a curvilinear P–V relationship, exhibiting an inflexion at low lung volume. The "minimal effective" PEEP corresponds to the opening pressure of recruitable lung areas, since it prevents distal airway collapse and restores FRC, without overdistending the recruited alveoli. When the level of PEEP is further augmented, the pattern of P–V curves is markedly affected: diminution of hysteresis, suppression of the inflexion on the ascending limb, and increase in compliance (Benito and Lemaire 1990) (Fig. 2). PEEP applied to a spontaneously breathing patient (CPAP) has the same beneficial effects on lung volume and compliance (Katz and Marks 1985).

Table 1. Functional residual capacity in patients with acute respiratory distress syndrome (ARDS)

	Year	n	FRC in l
MacIntyre	1970	5	1.120 + 0.16
Ramachandran and Fairlay	1970	10	1.20 + 0.4
Falke et al.	1972	7	1.48 + 0.78
Katz et al.	1981	8	1.5 + 0.2
Matamis et al.	1984c	12	0.90 + 0.25
Benito and Lemaire	1990	6	0.87 + 0.22 (27% pred.)

FRC, functional residual capacity

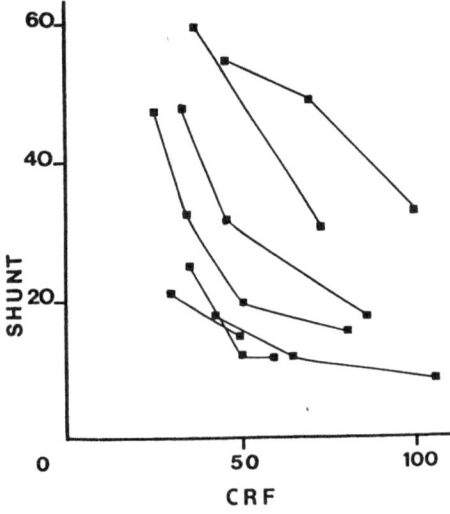

Fig. 1. Relationship of functional residual capacity (FRC) and shunt in seven ARDS patients at increasing levels of PEEP. FRC, which is markedly reduced at zero end expiratory pressure (ZEEP) (< 50% in every case), is increased stepwise by PEEP. At each increase of FRC there is a corresponding decrease of shunt. (From Matamis et al. 1984c)

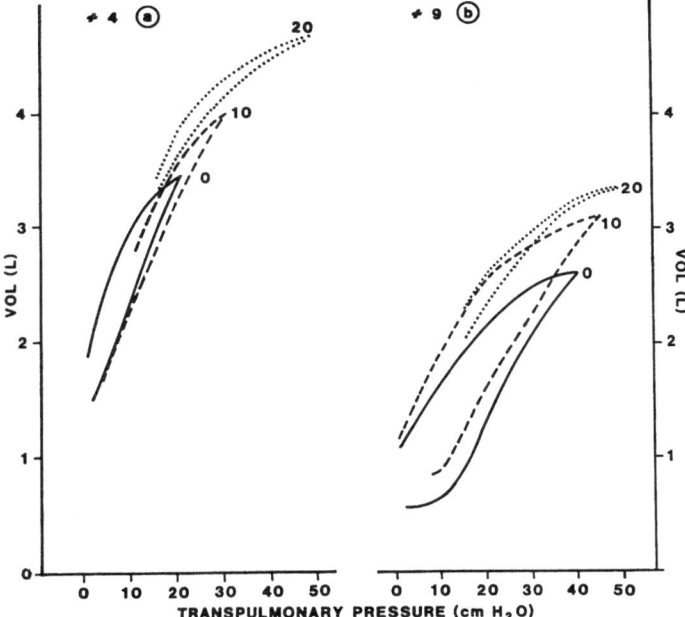

Fig. 2. Pressure-volume (P–V) curves traced with the 2-l syringe. *a* Patient no. 4, with normal lungs; *b* patient no. 9, with ARDS. The three P–V curves in each pannel correspond to different PEEP levels: 0, 10, and 20 cm H_2O. On the *left* (*a*): FRC is only slightly decreased (patient supine and curarization), compliance is normal, hysteresis reduced. On the *right* (*b*): FRC is reduced (0.5 l), hysteresis is increased, and there is an inflexion pressure on the ascending limb of the curve. When 20 cm H_2O PEEP is added, end expiratory lung volume is augmented, hysteresis reduced, and the inflexion on the ascending curve disappears. (From Benito and Lemaire 1990)

Gattinoni et al. (1987) recently compared, in ARDS patients, P–V curves and morphological data obtained from computed tomographic (CT) scans of the lung at increasing levels of PEEP. As lung pathology appeared extremely heterogeneous, with juxtaposition of normally aerated and dense areas, alveolar recruitment induced by PEEP also appeared unevenly distributed with the opening of some recruitable parenchyma, but no effect on the non-aerated tissue, and overdistension of the normally aerated zones. Alveolar recruitment was found to be linearly correlated with the ratio of inflation compliance to starting compliance (Cinf/Cstart), emphasizing the clinical relevance of the inflexion pressure. Whether diffuse or localized, the alveolar recruitment is usually obvious on plain chest X-ray, as both lungs appear definitely more aerated when enough PEEP is applied.

Where does the apparently dislodged alveolar edema go? Examining lung pathology in dogs with oleic acid-induced edema, Malo et al. (1984) have elegantly shown that application of PEEP mobilized the fluid from the alveolar space to the interstitium, especially the peribronchial and perivascular areas.

Hemodynamics

Soon after introduction of the clinical induction of PEEP it was observed that the increase in intrathoracic pressure reduced the cardiac output. This effect was first described by Cournand et al. as early as 1948.

The main factor responsible for the decreased cardiac output is the reduction of biventricular preload, due to the decrease of venous return. Most often, ventricular telediastolic volumes are reduced by PEEP ventilation. Viquerat et al. (1983) demonstrated in ten ARDS patients, that a 12-cm H_2O PEEP reduced the cardiac output by an average of 14%, the left ventricular end-diastolic (LVED) volume from 56 to 48 ml/m^2, and the right ventricular end-diastolic volume (RVED) from 83 to 75 ml/m^2. Similarly, Dhainaut et al. (1986) measured a 25% decrease of both ventricular volumes when 20 cm H_2O PEEP was applied, the ejection fraction remaining unchanged.

Qvist et al. (1975), in dogs with oleic acid-induced pulmonary edema, and Dhainaut et al. (1986), in patients with ARDS, showed that plasma volume expansion could reestablish ventricular volumes and cardiac output to control values. Such a preload reduction has been frequently overlooked in the past because of the misleading increase in intravascular pressure induced by PEEP. Computing the transmural left and right atrial pressures (by subtracting the esophageal pressure) actually gives a closer estimation of ventricular filling pressures (Qvist et al. 1975).

In a few studies, the right ventricle (RV) was shown to dilate markedly during PEEP ventilation (Hurford et al. 1986). Neidhart and Suter (1988), measuring the thermal RV ejection fraction of 11 ARDS patients, showed that PEEP induced a 25% increase of the RVED volume. Martin et al. (1987) documented a similar RV enlargement during PEEP in 2 of 13 patients. RV dilation may compress the left ventricle (LV), reduce its diastolic compliance, and increase LVED pressure. Using echocardiography, Jardin et al. (1981) demonstrated a septal "shift" at high level of PEEP (30 cm H_2O). The cause of RV dilation, which occurs only in some patients, is not very clear. Perhaps it is due to associated myocarditis in viral pneumonias, or right coronary compression, or unusually increased pulmonary vascular resistance (Hurford et al. 1986).

A substantial decrease of cardiac output due to PEEP only occurs when pulmonary compliance is normal or merely slightly reduced. In patients with severe ARDS, and a markedly reduced compliance, the hemodynamic effects of PEEP appear limited. This "shield effect" has been attributed to the coexistence of large shunts, protecting a noticeable part of pulmonary circulation from high alveolar pressure and collapse.

Gas Exchange

Intrapulmonary Shunt

Re-opening of edematous and collapsed alveoli is the basic effect of PEEP ventilation. Falke et al., as early as 1972, reported a linear relationship between the increase of PaO_2 and lung volumes during PEEP. Augmentation of the lung available for gas exchange decreases the intrapulmonary shunt. Examination of the pulmonary P–V curves provides a good predictor of the airway pressure at which alveolar recruitment occurs. The increase of lung volume does not vary linearly with the level of PEEP when it is increased stepwise, but occurs abruptly beyond a given threshold, called "opening pressure."

Besides alveolar recruitment, the decrease of cardiac output is obviously the second main mechanism for the improvement of intrapulmonary shunt during PEEP (Dantzker et al. 1980), according to the well-established linear relationship

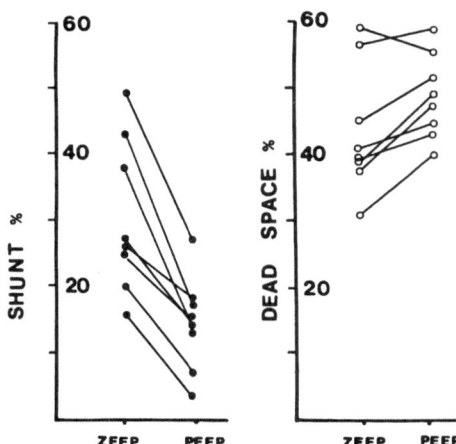

Fig. 3. Effects of PEEP on gas exchange in eight ARDS patients. Cardiac output decrease due to PEEP has been corrected by dopamine infusion. However, shunt is decreased and dead space increased (both were measured using the multiple inert gas elimination technique). (From Matamis et al. 1984b)

between shunt and cardiac output (Lemaire et al. 1976). However, Brun-Buisson et al. (1987) demonstrated that this effect contributed significantly to the decrease in shunt only in those patients ventilated at levels of PEEP higher than the "inflexion" pressure, or with no inflexion on P–V curves. Moreover, the support of cardiac output by plasma volume expansion or dopamine infusion (Hemmer et al. 1980; Matamis et al. 1984a) does not suppress the PEEP-induced shunt reduction. Therefore, the decrease in cardiac output is not a prerequisite for the reduction of shunt in most patients (Fig. 3).

PaO_2—TaO_2

The expected improvement of PaO_2 with PEEP is entirely attributed to the decrease of intrapulmonary blood shunting. However, when cardiac output is severely depressed by PEEP, the associated decrease of $P\bar{v}O_2$ may result in a decreased PaO_2, even if the shunt is diminished. Accordingly, the ultimate goal of PEEP therapy cannot be merely to decrease the shunt, especially at the expense of cardiac output, but should be to increase oxygen delivery ($TaO_2 = CI \times CaO_2$) to tissues, which is predominantly influenced by the cardiac output, and is decreased with it. In the study by Suter et al. (1975), "best PEEP" was also defined as the PEEP level at which TaO_2 was highest. There is now a considerable interest in the relationship between oxygen consumption ($\dot{V}O_2$) and oxygen transport (TaO_2) in ARDS patients, particularly with respect to PEEP-induced variations of cardiac output, as several recent studies have suggested a pathological dependency of $\dot{V}O_2$ on TaO_2 in such patients, occurring above the (low) range of TaO_2 where a physiological dependency occurs (Danek et al. 1980; Bihari et al. 1987; Mohsenifar et al. 1983; Shoemaker et al. 1988).

These findings support the concept of an oxygen debt in such patients, which could be responsible for tissue hypoxia at levels of TaO_2 well within the normal range, and ultimately responsible, at least in part, for the development of multiple organ failure. Using an increase "oxygen flux test" by infusing prostacyclin in patients with acute respiratory failure (ARF) and sepsis, Bihari et al. (1987) were thus able to unmask such an oxygen debt, with an increased $\dot{V}O_2$ following the increased TaO_2, in the most severe patients who eventually died, whereas no such increase in $\dot{V}O_2$ was found in nonfatal disease or normal controls. Likewise, Shoemaker et al. (1988) showed that survival was improved in postoperative patients in whom TaO_2 was increased towards supranormal levels, as compared with patients in whom standard therapy was applied, with no attempt at "optimizing" TaO_2.

However, methodological problems remain to be settled before such conclusions may be accepted as valid. A basic problem is the method used for comparing $\dot{V}O_2$ and TaO_2 in such studies, where $\dot{V}O_2$ is not measured, but calculated from CI and $(a-\bar{v})CO_2$, introducing a common variable (CI) in both calculations of $\dot{V}O_2$ and TaO_2; in such case, $\dot{V}O_2$ and TaO_2 will invariably be found to be correlated by mathematical coupling. It is interesting to note that, in studies where $\dot{V}O_2$ has been measured independently from TaO_2, the former was found to vary independently from the latter—or rather not to change at all—when cardiac output varied within the physiological range (e.g., following the application of PEEP) (Annat et al. 1986; Pepe and Culver 1985).

Nevertheless, patients with overtly reduced tissue perfusion, such as patients with lactic acidosis, obviously benefit from an increased TaO_2 and demonstrate an increased $\dot{V}O_2$ following volume expansion or the administration of an inotropic agent to increase tissue perfusion and oxygen transport (Gilbert et al. 1986). Obviously, PEEP should be applied cautiously in patients with evidence of decreased tissue perfusion, and monitoring of cardiac output is necessary in such cases.

CO_2 Elimination—Dead Space

Elimination of CO_2 is improved by the $\dot{V}a/Q$ homogenization due to PEEP. However, this is usually not apparent clinically because PEEP induces a substantial increase of dead space: the reduction of capillary flow increases alveolar dead space, and the anatomical dead space is also increased because of tracheal and bronchial dilation.

Matamis et al. (1984a) reported in eight patients with ARDS that a 17 cm H_2O PEEP increased the physiologic dead space by 10%, while cardiac output was maintained by a dopamine infusion. Suter et al. (1975) showed by increasing the level of PEEP in ARDS patients that VD/VT first decreased (presumably due to alveolar recruitment), had its lowest value at "best PEEP," and increased when the PEEP level was augmented further, due to alveolar overdistension. Accordingly, variations of end-tidal PCO_2 have been used for PEEP titration (Blanch et al. 1987).

Complications

Hemodynamics

We have already mentioned the possible deleterious influence of the cardiac output drop on PaO_2 via a $P\bar{v}O_2$ decrease and the oxygen delivery. In addition, the reduction of several regional specific blood flows—to the brain, heart, kidney, and liver—may be of clinical importance. Correction of PEEP-induced hemodynamic alterations is therefore mandatory. Plasma volume expansion and inotropic drug infusion are commonly used in the most severe patients, when no spontaneous breathing is possible (sedation, paralysis). Likewise, inermittent mandatory ventilation (IMV) was first introduced by Kirby et al. (1975) to alleviate the deleterious hemodynamic effects of high level PEEP, spontaneous breaths yielding a decrease of intra thoracic pressure.

Right heart catheterization, using a Swan-Ganz balloon tipped pulmonary artery catheter, is indicated in patients with severe ARDS ventilated with PEEP levels higher than 10 cm H_2O. This makes it possible to monitor filling pressures and cardiac output and also—in view of the great interest in sampling mixed venous blood—allows computation of $(a-\bar{v})O_2$ difference, $\dot{V}O_2$ and venous admixture or shunt. The value of pulmonary artery occluded pressure (PAOP) with high levels of PEEP has repeatedly been questioned. Teboul et al. (1989) showed recently that, in patients with severe ARDS, the PAOP remained identical to LVEDP, even at PEEP levels as high as 20 cm H_2O. The potentially dangerous maneuver of disconnecting a patient temporarily in order to measure PAOP is useless and misleading and thus should be completely abandoned.

Barotrauma

Pneumothorax is a common event during the course of ARDS, probably more common when PEEP is used. Besides large pleural air collection, localized tension pneumothorax—usually mediastinal—has been described (Gobien et al. 1982). Due to inability of the ARDS lung to collapse, there is usually no major displacement of the mediastinum, heart, and/or diaphragm. Instead, these localized pneumothorax present as loculated paracardiac or subphrenic air collection. They are best disclosed by CT scanning which is used more and more in ICU patients. These localized air collections are frequently poorly tolerated and can produce a gaseous tamponade. Drainage may be difficult.

Barotrauma may have other aspects. Churg et al. (1983) described three cases of ARDS in which lungs became hyperlucent, with scattered cystic foci. All three patients had been ventilated with high levels of PEEP and high FiO_2. Whether this is a particular form of interstitial emphysema, as reported by Pratt et al. (1979) in the morphological study of the ECMO project, remains debated. Some etiologies are preferentially encountered in such cases, such as acute pulmonary vasculitis (Schlemmer et al. 1988) and paraquat intoxication (Lemaire et al. 1982). A different form of lung cavitation is due to aseptic infarcts, as reported by Redline et al. (1985) and Jones et al. (1985).

Recently, several authors showed that hyperventilation could induce severe alveolar edema (see Gattinoni, in Chap. 7). Dreyfuss et al. (1988) demonstrated that the deleterious effect of hyperventilation was more related to lung volume augmentation than to increased airway pressure. Application of PEEP certainly increases airway and intrathoracic pressures. The influence on alveolar pressure may be especially important (and deleterious) in case of inhomogeneous lung (Gattinoni et al. 1985). This concept induced implementation of other forms of mechanical ventilation, less responsible for barotrauma: inverted I/E ratio and pressure controlled (see Andersen in Chap. 10), PRV (see Räsänen in Chap. 7), and $ECCO_2R$ (see Gattinoni in Chap. 9).

Extravascular Lung Water

Despite the improvement in blood gases and X-ray clearing induced by PEEP, extravascular lung water is not reduced. Alveolar fluid is actually redistributed within the lung. Due to lymphatic compression and interstitial pressure increase, the total amount of extravascular lung water is increased (Rizk and Murray 1982).

Besides this local, purely mechanical effect, PEEP ventilation causes sodium and water retention by hemodynamic and hormonal mechanisms. Hemmer et al. (1980) and Annat et al. (1983) demonstrated that application of PEEP reduced urinary output and sodium excretion, and simultaneously induced an augmentation of urinary levels of ADH. This was accompanied by an increase in plasma renin activity (Annat et al. 1983). Another determinant of sodium and water retention is probably the reduction of renal blood flow. More recently, Andrivet et al. (1988) measured a reduction of plasma atrial natriuretic factor during PEEP ventilation, related to right atrial transmural pressure—and probably volume—decrease. Whatever the mechanisms, water and sodium retention is a common event during PEEP ventilation, and fluid balance should accordingly be carefully monitored.

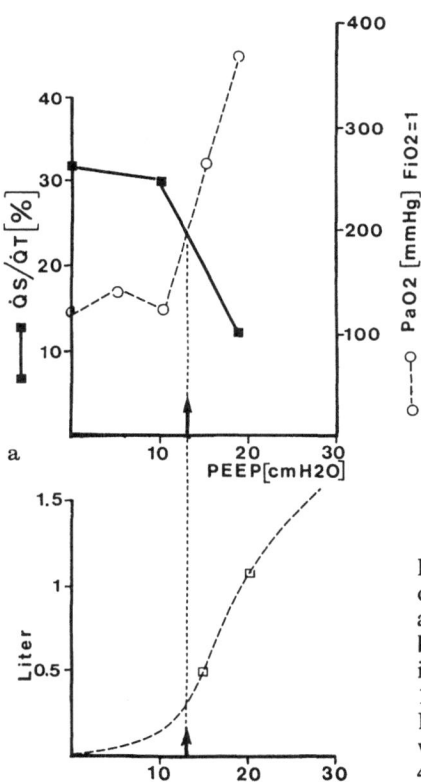

Fig. 4 a, b. Inflexion pressure and gas exchange during PEEP ventilation. **a** PaO$_2$ and venous admixture ($\dot{Q}S/\dot{Q}T$) as a function of PEEP. **b** P–V curve (PAW, airway pressure; volume in liters). An inflexion is clearly depicted at 14 cm H$_2$O. When PEEP is lower than 14 cm H$_2$O, no effect is seen on PaO$_2$ or shunt; when PEEP is 20 cm H$_2$O, PaO$_2$ reaches 400 mmHg and $\dot{Q}S/\dot{Q}T$ drops drastically to 12%. (From Matamis et al. 1984b)

Titration of PEEP

Titration of PEEP has been the subject of much debate during the past 15 years. The ultimate goal is to determine the adequate level of airway pressure that will sufficiently improve gas exchange with the least possible deleterious hemodynamic effects. At the bedside, the measurement of thoracopulmonary compliance can provide, non-invasively, the level of airway pressure at which alveolar recruitment is likely to occur. "Effective" compliance may be used (Suter et al. 1975), as well as P–V curve tracings using a 2-l syringe (Benito and Lemaire 1990). Patients with flat P–V curves (no inflexion) usually do not respond to PEEP or exhibit a decreased shunt via a reduction of cardiac output (Abrouk 1988). Titration of PEEP using the expired CO_2 proved to be similarly efficient (Blanch et al. 1987). In patients with ARDS of mild to moderate severity, aiming to obtain reasonable levels of PaO_2 (and/or of transcutaneous SaO_2), allowing reduction of FiO_2 with no decrease in blood pressure and urinary output is certainly an acceptable strategy. It is only in the most severe forms of respiratory failure that hemodynamic monitoring and a precise determination of the "optimal" PEEP level are necessary (Fig. 4).

References

Andrivet P, Adnot S, Brun-Buisson C, Chabrier E, Darmon JY, Braquet P, Lemaire F (1989) Involvement of ANF in the acute antidiuresis during PEEP ventilation. J Appl Physiol 65:1967–1975

Annat G, Viale JP, Bui Xuan B, Aissa OH, Benzoni D, Vincent M, Gharib C, Motin J (1983) Effect of PEEP ventilation on renal function, plsma renin, aldosterone, neurophysins and urinary ADH and prostaglandins. Anesthesiology 58:136–141

Annat G, Viale JP, Percival C, Fromant M, Motin J (1986) Oxygen delivery and uptake in the adult respiratory distress syndrome. Am Rev Respir Dis 133:999–1001

Ashbaugh DG, Bigelow DB, Petty TL, Levine BE (1967) Respiratory distress in adults. Lancet 2:319–323

Benito S, Lemaire F (1990) Mechanical P–V relationship in acute respiratory distress syndrome in adults: role of PEEP. J Crit Care 5:27–34

Bihari D, Smithies M, Gimson A, Tinker J (1987) The effects of vasodilation with prostacyclin on oxygen delivery and uptake in critically ill patients. N Engl J Med 317:397–403

Blanch L, Fernandes R, Benito S, Mancebo J, Net A (1987) Effect of PEEP on the arterial minus end-tidal carbon dioxide gradient. Chest 92:451–454

Brun-Buisson C, Abrouk F, Ben Lakhal S, Lemaire F (1987) Reduction of venous admixture with PEEP during human ARF. Respective role of alveolar recruitment vs decrease in blood flow (Abstr). Am Rev Respir Dis 135:A6

Churg A, Golden J, Fligiel S, Hogg JC (1983) Bronchopulmonary dysplasia in the adult. Am Rev Respir Dis 127:117–120

Cournand A, Motley HL, Werko L, Richards DW (1948) Physiological studies on the effects of intermittent positive pressure breathing on cardiac output in man. J Physiol 152:162–174

Danek SJ, Lynch JP, Weg JG, Dantzker DR (1980) The dependence of oxygen uptake on oxygen delivery in the adult respiratory distress syndrome. Am Rev Respir Dis 122:387–395

Dantzker Dr, Lynch JP, Weg JG (1980) Depression of cardiac output is a mechanism of shunt reduction in the therapy of acute respiratory failure. Chest 77:636–642

Dhainaut JF, Devaux JY, Monsallier JF, Brunet F, Villemant D, Huyghebaert MF (1986) Mechanisms of decreased left ventricular preload during continuous postive pressure ventilation in ARDS. Chest 90:74–80

Dreyfuss D, Soler P, Basset G, Saumon G (1988) High inflation pressure pulmonary edema. Respective effects of high airway pressure, high tidal volume and PEEP. Am Rev Respir Dis 137:1159–1164

Falke KJ, Pontoppidan H, Kumar A, Leith DE, Geffin B, Laver MB (1972) Ventilation with positive end-expiratory pressure in acute lung disease. J Clin Invest 51:2315–2323

Gattinoni L, Pesenti A, Avalli L, Rossi F, Bombino M (1987) Pressure-volume curve of total respiratory system in acute respiratory failure—a computed tomographic scan study. Am Rev Respir Dis 136:730–736

Gilbert EM, Haupt MT, Mandanas RY, Huaringa AJ, Carlson RW (1988) The effect of fluid loading blood transfusion and catecholamine infusion on oxygen delivery and consumption in patients with sepsis. Am Rev Respir Dis 134:837–878

Goblin RP, Reines HD, Schabel SI (1982) Localized tension pneumothorax. Unrecognized form of barotrauma in adult respiratory distress syndrome. Radiology 142:15–19

Hemmer M, Viquerat CE, Suter PM, Vollotton MB (1980) Urinary antidiuretic hormone excretion during mechanical ventilation and weaning in man. Anesthesiology 52:395–400

Hurford W, Barlai-Kovach M, Lynch K, Zapol WM, Strauss HW, Lowenstein E (1986) Effect of the ARDS and PEEP on bi-ventricular function (Abstract). Am Rev Respir Dis 133:A304

Jardin F, Farcot JC, Boisante L, Curien N, Margairaz A, Bourdarias JP (1981) Influence of positive end expiratory pressure on left ventricular performance. N Engl J Med 304:387–392

Jones R, Zapol WM, Thomashefski JF, Kirton OC, Kobayashi K Reid LM (1985) Pulmonary vascular pathology: human and experimental studies. In: Zapol WM, Falke KJ (eds) Acute respiratory failure. Dekker, New York, pp 23–146

Katz JA, Marks JD (1985) Inspiratory work with and without continuous positive airway pressure in patients with acute respiratory failure. Anesthesiology 63:598–607

Katz JA, Ozanne GM, Zinn SE, Fairley HB (1981) Time course and mechanisms of lung-volume increase with PEEP in acute pulmonary failure. Anesthesiology 54:9–16

Kirby RR, Downs JB, Civetta JM (1975) High level PEEP in acute respiratory insufficiency. Chest 67:156–163

Kumar A, Falke KJ, Geffin B, Aldredge CF, Laver MB, Lowenstein E, Pontoppidan H (1970) Continuous positive pressure ventilation in acute respiratory failure (effects on hemodynamics and lung function). N Engl J Med 283:1430–1436

Lemaire F, Harari A, Rapin M, Jardin F, Teisseire B, Laurent D (1976) Assessment of gas exchange during VA bypass using the membrane lung In: Zapol WM, Qvist J (eds) Academic, New York. Artificial lungs for acute respiratory failure. pp 421–422

Lemaire F, Cerrina J, Lange F, Harf A, Carlet J, Bignon J (1982) PEEP induced airspace overdistension complicating paraquat lung. Chest 81:654–657

Lutch JS, Murray JF (1972) Continuous positive pressure ventilation: effects on systemic oxygen transport and tissue oxygenation. Ann Intern Med 76:193–202

Malo J, Ali J, Wood CDH (1984) How does positive end-expiratory pressure reduce intrapulmonary shunt in canine pulmonary edema? J Appl Physiol 57:1002–1010

Marini JJ, Culver BH, Kirk W (1985) Flow resistance of exhalation valves and PEEP devices used in mechanical ventilation. Am Rev Respir Dis 131:850–854

Martin C, Saux P, Albanese J, Bonneru JJ, Gouin F (1987) Right ventricular function during positive end expiratory pressure. Thermodilution evaluation and clinical application. Chest 92:999–1004

Matamis D, Lemaire F, Harf A, Teisseire B, Brun-Buisson C (1984a) Redistribution of pulmonary blood flow induced by PEEP and dopamine infusion in ARF. Am Rev Respir Dis 129:39–44

Matamis D, Lemaire F, Harf A, Brun-Buisson C, Ansquer JC, Atlan G (1984b) Total Respiratory pressure volume curves in the adult respiratory distress syndrome. Chest 86:58–66

Matamis D, Lemaire F, Rieuf P (1984c) Augmentation de la capacité residuelle fonctionelle dans la ventilation en PEEP. Ann Fr Anesth Reanim 3:199–204

McIntyre RW, Law AK, Ramachandran PR (1970) Positive expiratory pressure plateau: improved gas exchange during mechanical ventilation. Can Anaesth Soc J 16:477–486

Mohsenifar Z, Golbach P, Tashkin DP, Campisi DJ (1983) Relationship between oxygen delivery and oxygen consumption in the adult respiratory distress syndrome. Chest 84:267–271

Neidhart PP, Suter PM (1988) Changes in right ventricular function during mechanical ventilation. Intensive Care Med Suppl 14:471–473

Pepe PE, Culver BH (1985) Independently measured oxygen consumption during reduction of oxygen delivery by PEEP. Am Rev Respir Dis 132:288–292

Pepe PE, Hudson LD, Carrico CJ (1984) Early application of PEEP in patients at risk for the ARDS. N Engl J Med 311:281–286

Pinsky MR, Hrehocik D, Culpepper JA, Snyder JV (1988) Flow resistance of expiratory positive pressure systems. Chest 94:788–791

Pratt PC, Vollmer RT, Shelburne JD, (1979) Pulmonary morphology in a multihospital collaborative extracorporeal membrane oxygenation project. Am J Pathol 95:191–208

Qvist JH, Pontoppidan H, Wilson RS, Lowenstein E, Laver MB (1975) Hemodynamic response to mechanical ventilation with PEEP. Anesthesiology 42:45–55

Ramachandran PR, Fairley HB (1970) Changes in functional residual capacity during respiratory failure. Can Anaesth Soc 17:359–369

Redline S, Thomashefski JF, Altose MD (1985) Cavitating lung infarction after bland pulmonary thromboembolism in patients with the ARDS. Thorax 40:915–919

Rizk N, Murray JH (1982) PEEP and pulmonary edema. Am J Med 72:381–383

Schlemmer B, Yana C, Boudjadja A, Frija F, Le Gall JR (1988) CT-scan patterns of interstitial pulmonary emphysema in adults during mechanical ventilation for ARDS (Abstr.) Intensive Care Med 14:265

Shoemaker WC, Appel PL, Kram HB (1988) Tissue oxygen debt as a determinant of lethal and nonlethal postoperative organ failure. Crit Care Med 16:1117–1120

Smith TC, Marini JJ (1988) Impact of PEEP on lung mechanics and work of breathing in severe airflow obstruction. J Appl Physiol 65:1488–1499

Spearman CB (1988) PEEP: terminology and technical aspects of PEEP devices and systems. Crit Care Med 33:434–443

Suter PM, Fairley HB, Isenberg MD (1975) Optimum end expiratory airway pressure in patients with acute pulmonary failure. N Engl J Med 292:284–289

Teboul JL, Brun-Buisson C, Zapol WM, Abrouk F, Rauss A, Lemaire F (1989) Comparison of left ventricular end-diastolic pressure with pulmonary arterial occluded pressure during PEEP in patients with severe ARDS. Anesthesiology 70:261–266

Tuxen DV (1989) Detrimental effect of PEEP during controlled mechanical ventilation of patients with severe airflow obstruction. Am Rev Respir Dis 140:5–9

Viquerat CE, Righetti A, Suter PM (1983) Biventricular volumes and function in patients with ARDS ventilated with PEEP. Chest 83:509–514

Intermittent Mandatory Ventilation

D. R. G. Browne and K. J. Falke

Historical Perspective

The term intermittent mandatory ventilation (IMV) was first used by Klein in 1973 (Downs et al. 1973) to describe a type of mechanical ventilation which enabled the intubated patient to breathe spontaneously in between mandatory tidal volumes delivered by the ventilator at a preset rate. The machine rate could be reduced over a period of time enabling the patient to perform an increasing part of the minute ventilation himself. This concept was developed from the successful use of continuous flow ventilation in the management of the respiratory distress syndrome of the newborn in 1971 (Kirby et al. 1971). Kirby et al. (1971) considered the ability to breathe spontaneously in between ventilator breaths in a continuous positive breathing circuit to be a considerable advance in the management of these infants. This concept had in fact been an inbuilt feature of some of the original Engstrom and Emerson ventilators, and as Benzer (1982) commented the principle had been used for many years during general anaethesia with manual squeezing of the bag to assist spontaneous breaths.

The technique of IMV was developed by Downs et al. (1973) as a new approach to weaning adult patients from mechanical ventilation. They claimed that IMV decreased the complexity of equipment required for ventilatory support and that it lessened the need for conventional ventilatory weaning measurements to be made, thus enabling patients who failed such conventional criteria to be considered for an earlier start to the weaning process. These workers considered that this method had psychological benefits for the patient who was frightened of breathing on his own without mechanical support. This technique provided a more gradual transition from mechanical to spontaneous breathing, with positive end expiratory pressure/continuous positive airway pressure (PEEP/CPAP) if necessary, than the conventional T-piece "on/off" trials. They claimed that weaning time could be reduced by overcoming discoordinated patterns of breathing because regular intermittent mechnical inflations would not interfere with the proper sequence of muscular efforts. They also felt that IMV would allow the patient to determine his own minute ventilation and thus produce a more physiological $paCO_2$ for himself than mechanical ventilation alone (Kirby et al. 1972). This would help to avoid a respiratory alkalosis with all the associated problems, such as a reduction in cerebral blood flow (Kety and Schmidt 1946), reduction in cardiac output (Hewitt et al. 1973), hypokalaemia, and an increae in oxygen consumption (Khambatta and Sullivan 1973). This aspect of control of the $paCO_2$ and pH was considered to be particularly useful in weaning patients who were suffering from chronic obstructive pulmonary disease (Downs et al. 1974a).

In another study Downs et al. (1974b) evaluated the role of IMV in weaning patients suffering from acute respiratory failure using the maintenance of a pH greater than 7.30 as one of the main criteria for success. They claimed that the patients required a shorter period of mechanical support overall compared with controlled mechanical ventilation (CMV). They considered this to be associated with the fact that patients could start to wean when they were still unable to fulfil the criteria for a T-piece trial and that the avoidance of a respiratory alkalosis at the time of weaning resolved the problems of the patient trying to maintain a low $paCO_2$ when breathing on his own. The authors measured the oxygen consumption ($\dot{V}O_2$) as a means of assessing the work of breathing in patients undergoing IMV compared with CMV. They found the $\dot{V}O_2$ to be higher in patients who had received CMV compared with IMV and thought this could be partially explained by the undesirable alkalotic state that could arise during CMV.

In 1975, the use of IMV and PEEP in the management of flail chest was first reported by Cullen et al. (1975). This study concerned retrospective and prospective groups of patients undergoing ventilatory support with CMV and IMV. These workers claimed that the mean ventilatory support time necessary for patients treated with IMV and PEEP was significantly less than for those treated with CMV. They concluded that lung contusion, rather than the abnormal mechanics, was the major factor determining the need for ventilatory support and that once the contusion had been successfully treated with IMV/PEEP, their patients were able to wean in spite of a flail segment.

During the mid-1970s the role of IMV was firmly established in the management of infants with the respiratory distress syndrome. DeLemos and McLaughlin (1973) showed that the total ventilatory support time and duration of weaning were significantly reduced in those infants using IMV compared with those treated with CMV. Similar findings were documented by Fricker et al. (1980). In 1977, Kirby stated that the weaning procedure was unquestionably simplified in infants using IMV compared with standard techniques. He showed that using IMV, the arterial blood gases and pH were the only criteria required for assessment of the weaning process and this obviated the need for additional apparatus and more elaborate pulmonary function tests. He also reported that the infant who maintained adequate ventilation at an IMV rate of two breaths or less per minute could be extubated satisfactorily.

The effect of low rate intermittent mandatory ventilation on the pulmonary function of low-birth-weight infants has been shown to increase the functional residual capacity (Shutack et al. 1982). Similar effects with improvement in gaseous exchange have been reported by Boynton et al. (1984) when using a combination of high frequency oscillatory ventilation and intermittent mandatory ventilation in critically ill neonates.

In order to appreciate some of the potential benefits that might result from IMV, some of the physiological effects associated with positive pressure ventilation of the lungs compared with spontaneous respiration will now be outlined.

IMV and Organ Function

The physiological effects of spontaneous and mechanical ventilation on the regional intrapulmonary gas distribution in awake and anaesthetised, paralysed man have been well documented and reviewed by various workers, including Nunn (1961), Froese and Bryan (1974), Bynum et al. (1976), Rehder et al. (1977), and Jones (1977, 1987). Froese and Bryan (1974) found that during spontaneous ventilation, awake or anaesthetised, the dependent part of the diaphragm had the greatest displacement. In the paralysed subject, however, positive pressure ventilation displaced the superior part of the diaphragm rather than the dependent part, thus incresing lung volume areas that were already expanded rather than helping to re-expand the dependent zones. Neither PEEP nor large breaths could restore the diaphragm to its normal functional residual capacity (FRC) position and breathing pattern.

Mechanical ventilation may result in overdistention of the terminal bronchioles and such increased airway pressures could be made worse by PEEP, thus enhancing the risk of barotrauma (Bone et al. 1975), (Petersen and Baier 1983). This type of barotrauma is more common in the presence of acute respiratory distress syndrome (ARDS) (Petersen and Baier 1983) and chronic obstructive pulmonary disease (COPD) (Kumar et al. 1973). However, it is the presence of high peak airway pressures rather than the level of PEEP (Petersen and Baier 1983) or large tidal volumes (Bone et al. 1975) that are now thought to be the more important risk factors. The development of a new generation of ventilators with a pressure relief valve opening at a preset peak pressure had reduced this hazard (Boysen et al. 1979; Heenan et al. 1980; Hillman et al. 1986).

Positive pressure ventilation of the lungs has been reported to have adverse effects on the cardiovascular and renal systems and may decrease the cardiac output (Cournand et al. 1948; Watson et al. 1962; Colgan et al. 1971; Qvist et al. 1975). The effect of mechanical ventilation with PEEP may be markedly affected by pre-existing pulmonary vascular disease as shown by Trichet et al. (1975) Urinary output has been shown to be compromised by mechanical ventilation (Baratz et al. 1971; Khambatta and Baratz 1972) and PEEP exaggerates this effect (Kumar et al. 1974).

The concept of IMV, therefore, combining positive pressure ventilation with spontaneous breathing has the potential for obviating some of the unwanted side effects resulting from the raised intrathoracic and intrapulmonary pressures associated with positive pressure ventilation.

IMV Studies

Effects of IMV on Cardiopulmonary Function

IMV and the Lungs. It has been shown in experimental animals as well as clinically that arterial blood gases may be equally well maintained with IMV as with CMV using identical levels of PEEP, provided the IMV is tolerated satisfactorily (Steinhoff et al. 1982; 1984). In a single computer tomographic (CT) study, Gattinoni et al. (Personal communication) observed an impressive improvement in the distribution of aerated lung structure after changing from CMV with PEEP to spontaneous ventilation with CPAP (Fig. 1). This indicated that spontaneous ventilation with positive airway pressure was capable of abolishing the negative effects of CMV on the distribution of ventilation. However, studies showing that unwanted side effects of CMV with PEEP on the

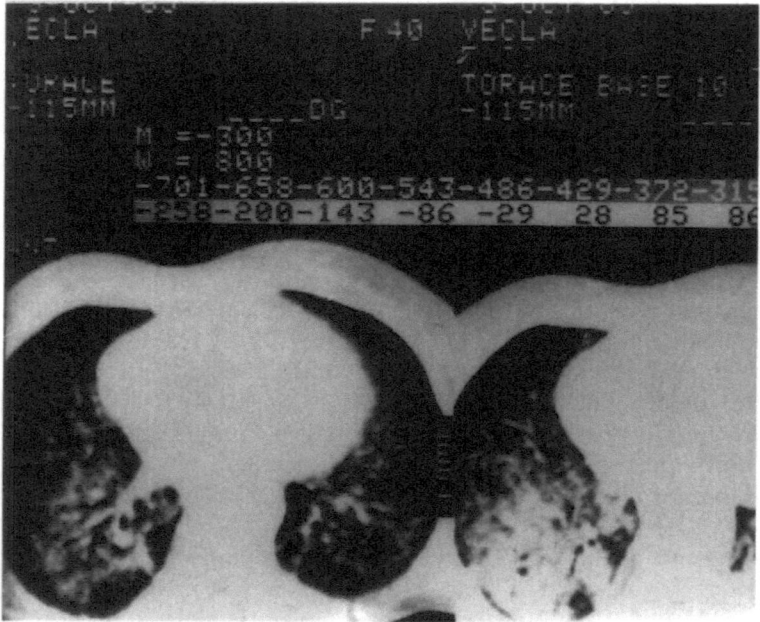

Fig. 1. Beneficial effect of spontaneous ventilation with continuous positive airway pressure (CPAP) in comparison to mechanical ventilation (CMV) with PEEP on the distribution of aerated lung structure. This shows a computer tomographe (CT) scan of the lungs from a patient with acute pulmonary disease during spontaneous breathing with CPAP (*left*) and shortly thereafter during CMV with PEEP (*right*) using similar tidal volumes and frequency as when breathing spontaneously. *Black structures* represent aerated and *white structures* nonaerated lung tissue. The distribution of nonaerated lung tissues on the *right* indicate basal infiltrates with maldistribution of ventilation. This is markedly improved if CPAP is used in conjunction with spontaneous breathing (*left*). (Courtesy of L Gattinoni)

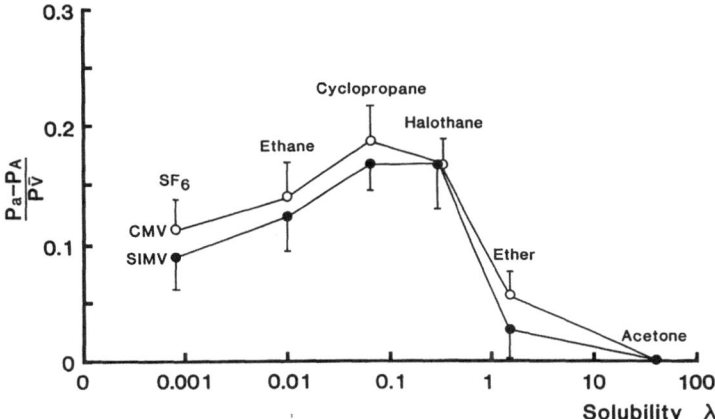

Fig. 2. Lack of significant improvement of the distribution of V_A/Q as obtained with the multiple inert gases elimination technique during SIMV if compared with CMV, both at the same level of PEEP (5 cm H_2O) in patients during weaning from postoperative mechanical ventilation. The inert gas elimination data are presented as the arterial-alveolar partial pressure differences normalized for the mixed partial pressures $(P_a - P_A)/P_{\bar{v}}$ plotted against the inert gas solubility λ. High values for the least soluble gases SF_6 and ethane reflect V_A/Q mismatch due to underventilated lung regions showing no significant improvement with SIMV. The diminished value for ether, however, documents an increase in dead space ventilation during SIMV. Both changes may become statistically significant with a larger group of patients (Santak et al. 1988)

distribution of ventilation/perfusion ratios ($\dot{V}A/\dot{Q}$) may be eliminated or reduced by a combination of spontaneous breathing and mechanical ventilation (IMV) are still lacking. In fact preliminary results of recent studies of the effect of IMV compared with CMV (both with 5 cm H_2O PEEP) on the distribution of $\dot{V}A/\dot{Q}$ using the multiple inert gases elimination technique in patients mechanically ventilated after major abdominal vascular surgery did not show a consistent improvement (Fig. 2) (Santak et al. 1988). Further studies under well-defined clinical conditions are necessary to clarify this problem.

IMV and the Heart. In 1975 Kirby et al. studied the cardiorespiratory effects of IMV with high levels of PEEP (20–25 cm H_2O) alternating with CMV and similar high levels of PEEP. Intravascular volume loading of the monkeys was performed throughout the study to protect against the haemodynamic responses to ventilation with PEEP as had been described by Qvist et al. (1975). Kirby et al. (1975) found that the cardiac output and mean aortic blood pressure were significantly depressed by periods of CMV when compared with periods of IMV. They concluded that high level PEEP was better tolerated with IMV than controlled ventilation under the same conditions in the monkeys they studied. In a further study on baboons which did not have intravascular volume loading, Zarins et al. (1977) tried to determine whether IMV and 20 cm H_2O CPAP offered any protection against PEEP-induced circulatory impairment with intermittent positive pressure ventilation (IPPV) and 20 cm H_2O PEEP. However, although they found the degree of cardiac output depression to be the same in both groups this could probably be accounted for by the high levels of PEEP used rather than the mode of ventilation.

In a further study on postoperative patients requiring mechanical ventilatory support, Downs et al. (1977) studied the ventilatory pattern, intrapleural pressures and the cardiac output to differentiate between the effects of PEEP and IPPV. They compared patients undergoing IMV (two breaths/min) using varying levels of PEEP with those undergoing IPPV without PEEP. These authors found that patients receiving IMV maintained their normal negative intrapleural pressures, atrial filling pressures and cardiac output in the presence of PEEP, unlike those receiving CMV. They concluded from this study that patients requiring mechanical ventilatory support could maintain better cardiopulmonary function when allowed to have some degree of spontaneous respiratory activity. They suggested that the spontaneous breaths would allow the intrapleural pressure to decrease sufficiently to maintain venous return, transmural cardiac filling pressure, cardiac output, and oxygen delivery at pre-PEEP levels without the necessity for intravascular volume loading.

Later work by Vuori and Klossner (1981) on postoperative cardiac patients revealed that the haemodynamics, oxygenation and oxygen consumption remained unchanged when patients were changed from a low rate of IMV (four breaths) with PEEP to spontaneous breathing with CPAP at the same level of PEEP. However, the authors suggested that more frequent mandatory breaths than four per minute might impair the haemodynamics similarly to that found with patients on CMV (Downs et al. 1977; Vuori et al. 1979). Studies in dogs by Venus et al. (1980) indicated that there was no significant difference in haemodynamic function in normal dogs undergoing IPPV compared with IMV and compared with spontaneous breathing (SB) but when PEEP was added the cardiac index decreased significantly. Steinhoff et al. (1984) also found there were no significant haemodynamic changes in enterally prehydrated dogs undergoing IMV compared with CMV both at 10 cm H_2O PEEP. In contrast, however, Mathru et al. (1982) revealed significant increases in the cardiac index of patients with normal left ventricular reserve when changed from CMV to IMV. In patients with poor left ventricular function, however, changing from CMV to IMV led to deleterious effects on the haemodynamic variables. They found these effects could be counteracted by using + 5 cm H_2O PEEP with the IMV.

A study by Simonneau et al. in 1982 compared the haemodynamic effects of CMV and PEEP with spontaneous breathing and CPAP both at 20 cm H_2O PEEP. They found that the cardiac index was significantly lower with CMV and PEEP compared with spontaneous breathing and CPAP. They concluded that the negative intrathoracic pressures associated with spontaneous inspiration reduced the need for aggressive levels of haemodynamic support when high levels of PEEP were needed to maintain oxygenation.

Chin et al. (1985) compared the effect of IMV on systemic oxygen consumption, systemic oxygen transport and tissue perfusion with that of CMV and with that of spontaneous breathing with CPAP using the same level of PEEP in patients suffering from pre-existing cardiopulmonary disease. They concluded that spontaneous breathing with CPAP provided for better systemic oxygen transport than either controlled ventilation or IMV with similar levels of PEEP. These workers attributed this beneficial effect to the higher cardiac index which they found in the spontaneously breathing group compared with the other two. However, there is no mention of the IMV rate in this study and this rate may be an important factor in determining the degree of reduction of cardiac output associated with the positive intrathoracic pressures produced by mechanical ventilation. An IMV rate of 12 breaths per minute would be more detrimental in this regard than an IMV rate of 4 breaths per minute. Similarly the setting of the trigger sensitivity with the demand valve may affect the cardiac output, although there are no such studies as yet. The less sensitive the machine, the more the negative intrathoracic pressure effects would be exaggerated.

In 1986 Wolff et al. (1986) investigated the effects of CMV with PEEP, IMV without PEEP and spontaneous breathing with CPAP in a group of patients who had undergone open heart surgery. Their findings showed that the cardiac output increased with IMV without PEEP compared with CMV with PEEP. The $\dot{V}CO_2$ and $\dot{V}O_2$ did not change when switching from IMV without PEEP to CPAP and they considered this indicated no difference in the work of breathing between the two systems. The FRC was found to be constant between CMV with PEEP and IMV without PEEP but was significantly reduced when breathing spontaneously with CPAP. The dead space ventilation was significantly reduced when breathing spontaneously compared with mechanical ventilation. These workers concluded from their studies that because IMV decreased the mean alveolar pressures and reduced dead space ventilation compared with CMV, it may be possible to start spontaneous breathing earlier with IMV than is usual in the recovery process. However, in the light of the study by Mathru et al. (1982) this effect may be beneficial only in the presence of normal left ventricular function.

Hastings et al. (1980) studied the cardiorespiratory dynamics in a group of postoperative cardiac patients in order to compare the process of weaning by IMV at the rate of four breaths per minute with weaning using the T-piece method. All patients were maintained 5 cm H_2O PEEP before weaning started and $+5$ cm H_2O CPAP when breathing spontaneously via the T-piece. These workers could find no improvement in the cardiac output in the IMV group compared with those patients breathing spontaneously with CPAP, nor was there any change in oxygen consumption or CO_2 production in either group during the weaning process. They concluded that they were unable to demonstrate any advantage to weaning by IMV and they recommended that spontaneous ventilation should be used for this purpose although they conjectured that the IMV mode was probably preferable in maintaining the cardiac output in hypovolaemic patients or those requiring high levels of PEEP as had been shown by Kirby et al. (1975) and Kirby et al. (1981). However, it could be argued that if these patients were able to wean satisfactorily breathing spontaneously on their own with a T-piece system, then there would be no indication to use any form of ventilatory support. Under these circumstances it would be inappropriate to try and establish any advantages of IMV when there was no need for it in the first place.

IMV and Discoordinated Patterns of Breathing

Discoordinated patterns of breathing associated with weaning from mechanical ventilation have been noted for many years (Chiang et al. 1973). One of the claims for IMV was that it could reduce the incidence of this respiratory muscle discoordination (Downs et al. 1973). Downs et al. (1973) and Downs et al. (1974b) argued that IMV minimised disuse atrophy of the respiratory muscles because the spontaneous breathing component would function as a graduated form of exercise. They also suggested that regular intermittent mechanical inflations in between periods spent breathing spontaneously would act to reinforce the proper sequence of muscular efforts for more efficient ventilation and so shorten weaning time. This hypothesis has been supported by Anderson et al. (1978, 1979). Other workers, however, have found that such discoordinated patterns of breathing and rapid respiratory rates were particularly associated with underlying problems, such as muscle fatigue (Cohen et al. 1982), inefficient gaseous exchange (Tobin et al. 1986), high central respiratory drives (Holle et al. 1982), and excessive ventilatory requirements resulting from the increased oxygen demands of the critically ill (Bursztein et al. 1978) and the increased CO_2 production from high glucose loads used in parenteral feeding (Askanazi et al. 1980; Herve et al. 1983; Laaban et al. 1985). Indeed, Herve et al. (1983) considered that problems associated with an increased CO_2 production in patients with compromised ventilatory function could be worsened during IMV. It has also been suggested that particular attention should be paid to treating any underlying nutritional deficiencies that could induce a myopathic state of the respiratory muscles which would render them more prone to fatigue (Gertz et al. 1977; Newman et al. 1977; Aubier et al. 1985). Once muscles show evidence of fatigue then it has been recommended that they should be rested if they are unable to cope with the work of breathing (Cohen et al. 1982; Rochester et al. 1977; Roussos and Macklem 1982; Rochester and Arora 1983; Braun 1984). IMV has made it possible to monitor the nonparalysed, relatively unsedated patient requiring ventilatory support more carefully. This has given the clinician access to a better understanding of the clinical status with the facility of increasing or decreasing the mechanical ventilatory component to suit the requirements of the patient more accurately.

Effects of IMV on Renal Function

In 1982 Steinhoff et al. published the results of a study comparing the renal effects of intermittent mandatory ventilation with those of controlled mechanical ventilation in patients suffering from acute respiratory failure. They found the urine flow and the osmolar and creatinine clearances to be significantly lower during 2-h periods of CMV compared with 2-h periods of IMV. They concluded that IMV should be used whenever possible in the management of acute respiratory failure in order to maintain renal function and to reduce water retention. In a further study in dogs it was shown that IMV was associated with a statistically improved urinary output and renal plasma flow (Steinhoff et al. 1984). They interpreted the improvement in renal function as being the consequence of decreased mean intrathoracic pressures during IMV as compared with CMV. However, the long-term effects of IMV or other forms of augmented ventilation on water and electrolyte balance or on renal function have not yet been studied in the clinical situation.

Effect of IMV on the Acid Base Status

One of the claims made for IMV by Downs et al. (1964b) was that it would obviate the respiratory alkalosis associated with the management of patients undergoing CMV. In recent years several workers have felt it would be more appropriate to compare the acid base changes associated with IMV and assist-controlled (triggered) mechanical ventilation (AMV) rather than CMV, as this AMV mode is more commonly used. In a study of patients who had undergone coronary artery bypass surgery, Hooper and Browning (1985) concluded that the AMV mode resulted in more respiratory alkalosis than IMV. They attributed these findings to the commonly increased respiratory rate associated with AMV and the addition of the extra machine-delivered tidal volumes with each breath. Hudson et al. (1985) hypothesised that during AMV patients might develop a respiratory alkalosis if they had a pathologically increased respiratory drive. Indeed, they found that in one such group with a respiratory alkalosis, IMV decreased the pH. They considered this decrease to be related to an increase in VCO_2 because it was not associated with any change in alveolar ventilation. The increase in VCO_2 was thought to reflect an increased work of breathing. This is in contrast to their findings in patients with head injuries who showed no decrease in pH when changed from AMV to IMV. These patients also had an increased VCO_2 but the pH remained unchanged because the alveolar ventilation increased to compensate. Such an increased respiratory rate under these circumstances could lead to ultimate fatigue of respiratory muscles in compromised patients. Similar results were obtained by Culpepper et al. (1985) who monitored respiratory rate and arterial blood gases in mechanically ventilated patients who underwent consecutive periods of AMV and IMV in randomised order. They concluded that AMV rarely produced a significant respiratory alkalosis on its own account and that any alkalosis occurring during such ventilation was the result of an abnormal respiratory drive that was only minimally influenced by the mode of ventilation be it assist-controlled or IMV. Therefore, in general, it may be said that it is preferable to avoid the rate of the machine being set by any abnormal rate of the patient and that this mechanical rate should always be set independently.

Technical Aspects of IMV

In order for IMV and CPAP systems to work correctly it is vitally important that constant positive airway and circuit pressures be supplied throughout the whole cycle of spontaneous inspiration and expiration. A sharp airway pressure drop during inspiration measured at the distal end of the endotracheal tube is a sign of either insufficient flow or added inspiratory resistance in the circuitry. According to studies by both Schlobohm et al. (1981) and Quan et al. (1981) such an inspiratory pressure drop may on its own account contribute to further deterioration of pulmonary function with a fall in the functional residual capacity and paO_2. In some instances it may be a sign of the increased respiratory drive

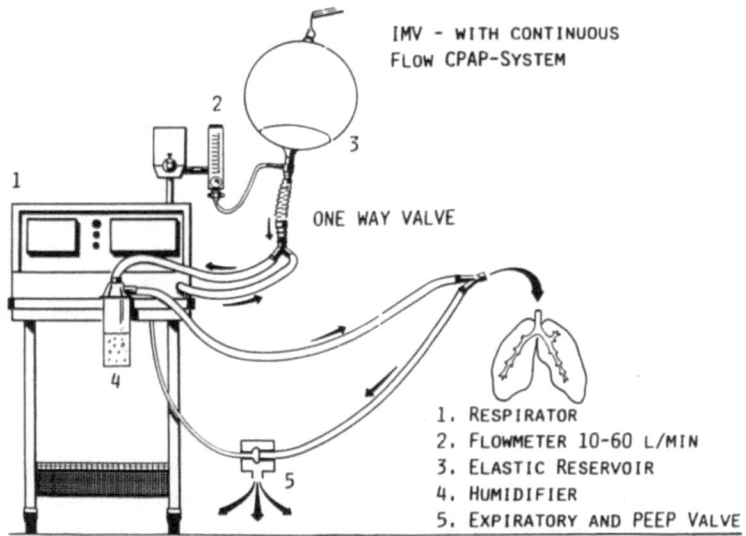

IMV - WITH CONTINUOUS FLOW CPAP-SYSTEM

ONE WAY VALVE

1. RESPIRATOR
2. FLOWMETER 10-60 L/MIN
3. ELASTIC RESERVOIR
4. HUMIDIFIER
5. EXPIRATORY AND PEEP VALVE

Fig. 3. Classical continuous flow IMV system. A continuous flow CPAP system is inserted into the inspiratory line of the respirator. During mechanical inspiration a one-directional valve prevents inspiratory gas from flowing backwards into the reservoir bag. The reservoir bag serves to stabilize inspiratory and expiratory airway pressures if the inspiratory flow demand exceeds the preset continuous flow rate. Sometimes, however, the continuous flow may have to be set close to the peak inspiratory flow demand of the patient (e.g., up to $45 \, 1 \times min^{-1}$ or more) in order to prevent a significant fall in inspiratory pressure as shown in the previous figure. Such high additional flow rates can only be adapted with safety for the patient if the machine is equipped with well-functioning high pressure relief valves and low resistant expiratory/PEEP valves. As far as the authors are aware such an IMV/CPAP has never been made available commercially by any European manufacturers to date

that is associated with inspiratory muscle fatigue and if this problem cannot be resolved by optimising the setting of the ventilator, pharmacological suppression of spontaneous breathing may be indicated.

IMV requires equipment which will allow the patient to continue to breathe spontaneously while mechanical breaths are superimposed intermittently. Throughout the process the patient should not be required to overcome external resistances which would involve an additional workload of breathing. These goals can be best accomplished by a continuous flow system. A humidified continuous gas flow of 15–25 l/min or more with the same F_1O_2 as set for mechanical ventilation is passed through the inspiratory limb of the ventilator circuit via a unidirectional valve. A pressurised reservoir bag of 5- to 25-l capacity is attached to the inspiratory limb of this continuous flow system in order to provide adequate inspiratory pressures should the peak inspiratory flow rate of the patient exceed the preset gas flow (Fig. 3). Additional requirements for a properly functioning system are as follows:

1. The trigger effort should be minimal in order to avoid detrimental respiratory effects with a reduction in FRC and increased work of breathing. The trigger sensitivity should therefore be set as high as possible, e.g., 0.5 mbar. This may not be possible on some machines because of inadvertent self-triggering.
2. Airway pressure should be monitored close to the airway in order to recognise and avoid detrimental negative pressure swings. Christopher et al. (1985) suggest that if the maximum negative pressure swing exceeds -4 cm H_2O or if it is greater than 30% of the negative inspiratory force at the beginning of inspiration, then the equipment should be modified.
3. PEEP should be maintained by continuous flow or activation of a demand valve.
4. All connections must be tightly secured.
5. The mechanical respiratory rate should be variable and range from high rates to zero.
6. Large bore tubing should be used throughout to avoid inspiratory and expiratory resistances.
7. Low-flow resistant, highly efficient humidifiers should be used, as well as low-flow resistant valves, particularly the PEEP valve (large bore tube under water is the best!).

One of the problems associated with a continuous flow system is the difficulty in measuring the expiratory volume of the patient. This is due to the presence of the relatively large continuous flow contaminating the gas volume expired by the patient.

More than a decade of clinical experience has shown that it is not necessary for the mechanical breaths to be synchronised with the spontaneous inspiratory efforts of the patient provided that the ventilator is equipped with a well-functioning pressure relief valve which will avoid any dangerous build-up of pressure should a mechanical breath be superimposed upon a spontaneous breath or cough. With a continuous flow system properly adjusted to the inspiratory flow demand of the patient, the pressure swings associated with spontaneous inspiration and expiration are very small. It would therefore be very difficult to synchronise individual mechanical breaths with the patient as substantial pressure swings below the preset end expiratory pressure level would be required to trigger the machine.

An alternative system for providing IMV incorporates the use of a demand valve. This system is the commonest type provided commercially at present, but it carries the inherent problem that the patient has to generate a certain amount of inspiratory force ("isovolaemic" inspiratory work) to open or "trigger" the demand flow valve before inhalation is possible. In some of the older models of ventilator, a substantial amount of added work was required with every single spontaneous breath in order to overcome the resistances in the circuit and to trigger the demand valve (Figs. 4, 5) (Samodelov and Falke 1988). Certain groups of patients with impaired thoracopulmonary mechanics involving a low FRC and poor compliance may have rapid respiratory rates which require such high peak inspiratory flow rates that it makes it impossible to tolerate IMV using these demand flow machines. This problem hampered the successful introduction of IMV in many institutions where continuous flow systems were never used. By using a spontaneously breathing lung model with mean inspiratory flow rates of 0.5 l/s, it has been shown that most of the more recently developed demand flow machines such as the Servo 900C, Puritan Bennett 7200, Draeger Eva and UV2 have lessened this problem. They provide conditions which allow the patient to inhale without having to generate additional inspiratory work compared with the

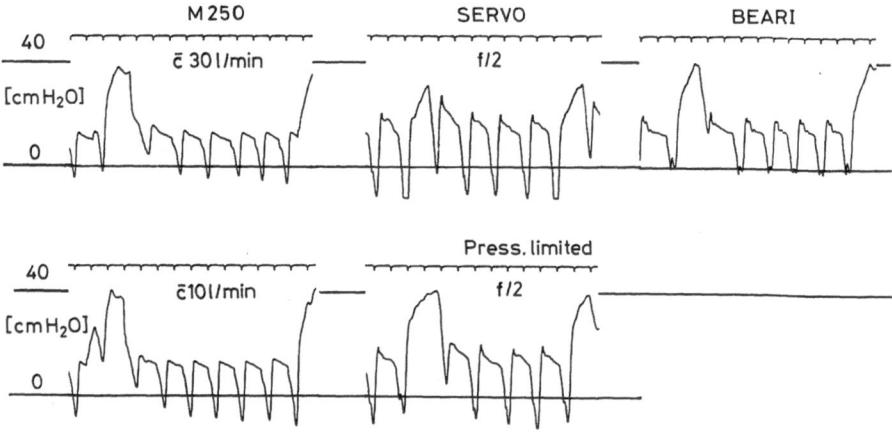

Fig. 4. Airway pressure tracings with different ventilators in the same patient showing that certain IMV/CPAP circuits fail to provide adequate conditions to match the requirements of the patient. The figure shows marked pressure swings below the preset PEEP level, indicating that the respirator does not supply the inspiratory flow needed during spontaneous inspiration and as a result of the ventilator circuit imposes an added inspiratory workload

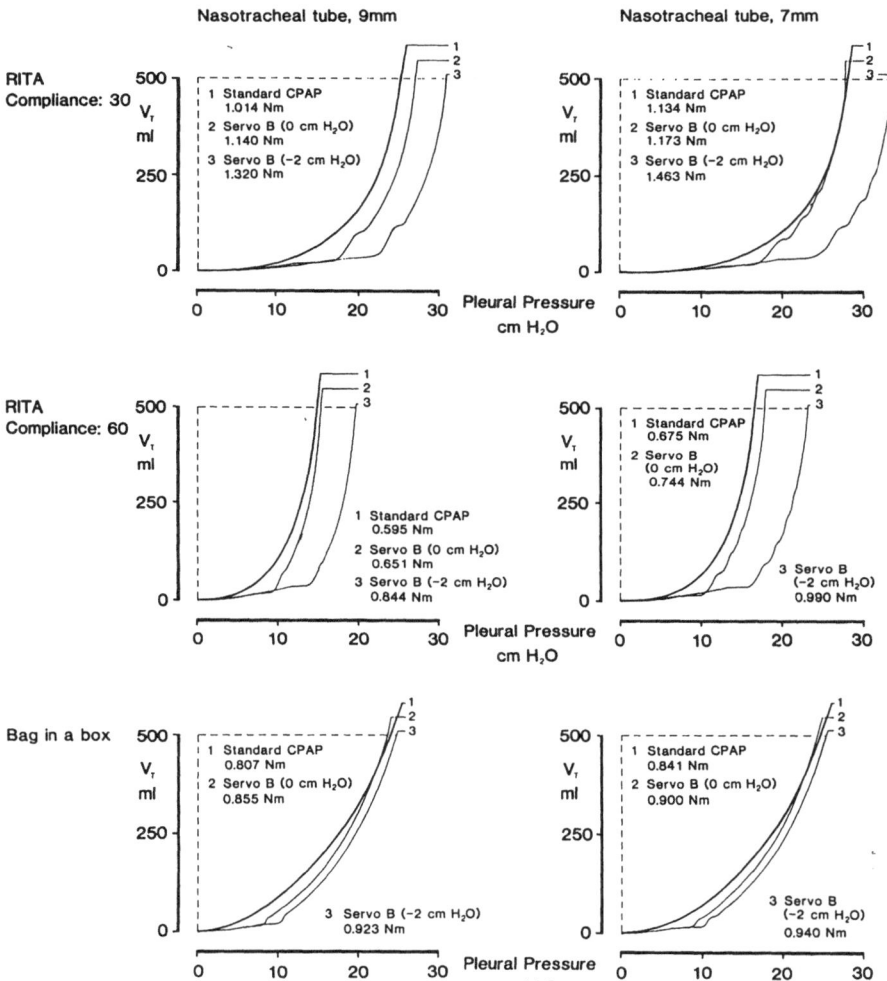

Fig. 5. Increased inspiratory work of breathing with the Siemens Servo B using two sizes of nasotracheal tubes. This shows the inspiratory work of breathing (*area encircled by inspiratory pressure volume curves and the dotted lines*) required during spontaneous inspiration accomplished with thorax-lung models (*RITA*) and a bag in the box circuit during a 500-ml breath with a sinusoidal flow wave taken within 1 s. The fat curve (*1*) represents the continuous flow CPAP reference system, the other curves (*2, 3*) the Siemens Servo B ventilator with different trigger sensitivities. Substantial increases in the work of inspiration associated with this particular demand flow system are demonstrated in this figure. Under these experimental conditions more modern ventilators such as the Servo C, the Bennett 7200, Draeger EVA and UV2 perform almost as well as the continuous flow system. (Samodelov and Falke 1988)

DEMANDFLOW (III)

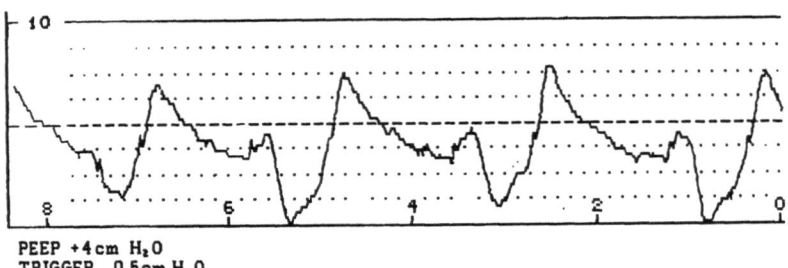

PEEP +4cm H₂0
TRIGGER 0.5cm H₂0

FLOW BY

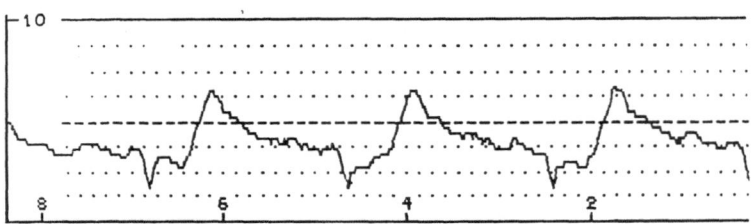

PEEP +4 cm H₂0
BASISFLOW 20 LpM
FLOW SENSIBILITY 1LpM

Fig. 6. Airway pressure tracings when breathing spontaneously to show reduction of negative pressure swings with flow-by compared with the demand-flow option. These results indicate that there was less inspiratory work for the patient to perform against external resistances using flow-by compared with the demand-flow option

continuous flow system. However, in order to achieve this goal a small amount of inspiratory pressure support (3–5 cm H_2O) must be activated and the trigger sensitivity must be set as high as possible (i.e., -0.5 to -1.0 mbar). Unfortunately, however, in the clinical setting this may lead to "self-triggering" occasionally associated with chaotic malfunctioning of the ventilator. Furthermore, self-triggering may be induced by small leaks in the circuit and this is more likely in the presence of high PEEP levels.

One of the methods currently being used to overcome any undesirable added inspiratory work is the concept of "inspiratory pressure support" (Brach et al. 1976; Kanak et al. 1985; MacIntyre 1986; Brochard et al. 1987; Samodelov and Falke 1988). In contrast to continuous flow systems, inspiratory pressure support—which is only available in conjunction with demand valve systems—eliminates the inspiratory work required to overcome the resistance of the endotracheal tube (Brochard et al. 1988). Although the inspiratory effort of the patient is minimised using this technique, pressure support still involves elements of time delay between the patient taking a breath and the circuitry filling up with gas to the predetermined level (2–5 cm H_2O pressure). Thus, in spite of considerable technical improvements in the demand flow systems, these outstanding problems have led to the development of a continuous "flow system" which is now commercially available on the Puritan Bennett 7200 and is known as Flow-by. This device is an attempt to combine the advantages of both continuous and demand flow systems. Flow-by causes the pneumatic system of the ventilator to deliver a predetermined flow of gas into the circuit prior to inspiration and the excess gas flow exits through the expiratory valve. Fresh gas is thus available to the patient as soon as an inspiratory effort is initiated and negative pressure swings associated with spontaneous inspiration have been shown to be reduced using this mode (Fig. 6). Flow-by also minimises the time delay between the inspiratory effort of the patient and the supply of gas to the Y-piece. However, the usefulness of this option remains to be established by appropriate studies.

In summary, modern mechanical IMV-type ventilators have reached a high standard for the optimal mechanical support of a spontaneously breathing patient. However, because of the complexity of these systems they are more prone to malfunction but it is hoped that these problems will soon be resolved by further advances in ventilator technology.

IMV Today

The IMV Concept

The multiplicity of techniques and modes of ventilatory support requires a simplified concept of clinical application. In principle there are three modes of ventilation which can be used in conjunction (or not) with PEEP or CPAP:

1. SV, spontaneous ventilation.
2. IMV, intermittent mandatory/mechanical ventilation.
3. CMV, controlled mechanical ventilation.

If the mechanical ventilator is always set in the IMV mode, then all three modes of ventilation can be easily achieved just by turning the mechanical ventilatory rate up and down. For SV with CPAP the rate is set at zero. CMV is obtained if the respiratory drive of the patient ceases due to appropriate alveolar ventilation and lung expansion or, if necessary, by giving respiratory depressant drugs or muscle relaxants.

A separate option for assisted mechanical ventilation (AMV) may be desirable in a few cases but it is not obligatory because conditions almost equal to AMV can be obtained by increasing the IMV rate. If the patient is fully ventilated by the machine, then this is called "total ventilatory support" (TVS), while if a substantial part of the ventilation is performed by the patient breathing spontaneously, then this is called "partial ventilatory support" (PVS) (Shapiro and Cane 1984). In adults, the rate of eight breaths per minute has been suggested as an arbitrary dividing line between TVS and PVS (Shapiro and Cane 1984). In practise, the degree of mechanical support will range from zero breaths/min with the patient breathing spontaneously totally on his own, to 12–20 breaths/min with the complete cessation of spontaneous breathing aided if necessary by pharmacological means. The optimum level of mechanical ventilatory support by IMV should match the ventilatory reserve of the patient.

In principle, the adequacy of partial ventilatory support is judged according to the established clinical and physiological criteria similar to the criteria for successful weaning. Among these the following must be included:

1. Absence of clinical signs of respiratory muscle fatigue such as a tachypnoea or discoordinated breathing patterns (Cohen et al. 1982).
2. A pH 7.32 or more and a $paCO_2$ less than 55 mm Hg.
3. Absence of a negative trend in arterial blood gases.
4. Absence of signs of sympathetic stimulation and cardiocirculatory symptoms.

Up until now there have been no major studies of respiratory muscle fatigue during partial ventilatory support. Methods for diagnosing this problem are being developed. The first results of the measurement of tracheal occlusion pressure utilising the trigger function of a demand flow machine to indicate respiratory muscle fatigue are already available (Herrera et al. 1985; Taylor et al. 1987). Because of the inherent problems of insufficient mechanical ventilatory support during the IMV process, patients must always be considered to be under weaning conditions and close bedside monitoring by the medical and nursing personnel is obligatory.

It remains a controversial issue whether patients who exhibit symptoms of inspiratory muscle fatigue should be weaned continuously by IMV or discontinuously by weaning trials interposed with phases of CMV putting the inspiratory muscles temporarily to complete rest. The latter technique has been found to be beneficial in certain COPD patients (Rochester et al. 1977; Marino and Braun 1982). However, it is unknown at present which approach is the more applicable to patients with acute respiratory failure who do not have a significant component of chronic lung disease.

Advantages and Disadvantages Claimed for IMV

Compared with CMV (Luce et al. 1981; Weisman et al. 1983)

Advantages

1. Has ability to match the appropriate amount of ventilatory support to suit the requirements of the patient.
2. Reduces the adverse effects of positive pressure ventilation with PEEP on circulatory and renal function.
3. Reduces the need for pharmacological interference (sedatives, relaxants).
4. Improved assessment of clinical status.

5. Allows a more gradual transition from high mean airway pressures to more normal ones in the weaning process.
6. Facilities an earlier start to a more controlled weaning process.
7. Maintains respiratory muscle function.
8. Avoids "fighting" the ventilator.
9. Is more acceptable to the patient psychologically.

Disadvantages

1. Risk of inadequate ventilatory support in the presence of infection, toxaemia, malnutrition, metabolic disturbances, compromised ventilatory function or high central ventilatory drive from the CNS.
2. Potential dangers of cardiac decompensation during weaning in patients with poor left ventricular function.
3. Increased work of breathing with malfunctioning equipment.
4. Difficulty in measurement of expired gas volumes with continuous flow systems.

A number of these points have already been discussed in detail earlier, but some demand repeated emphasis. The disadvantages listed all have potentially lethal consequences if not immediately identified by the clinical staff at the bedside. Thus, one of the original claims that IMV may lessen the need for ventilatory monitoring (Downs et al. 1973) is fraught with danger and is without foundation in the clinical setting. Indeed, it may be argued that one of the major advantages of IMV in clinical practise is that more frequent monitoring of a wider range of variables in the unparalysed, unsedated patient can alert the clinician to underlying problems. This will enable him to prescribe appropriate treatment earlier and match the correct amount of ventilatory support to suit the particular requirements of the patient at that time.

Conclusion

The advent of IMV has enabled the clinician to monitor the clinical status of the patient during the recovery process in a more elegant manner and to increase or decrease the ventilatory component as the clinical condition demands. This facility requires increased vigilance by the medical and nursing personnel in order to anticipate underlying problems which may be revealed by this technique and to avert disaster in a patient who may show signs of failing the challenge at any time. Indeed, management may be made more difficult in the presence of inexperienced staff. The future, however, may well show that IMV should be regarded as the basic setting for the ventilator in the management of patients requiring ventilatory support. This should range from FVS to PVS until the underlying clinical problems are resolved and the patient can breathe satisfactorily on his own.

References

Andersen JB, Kann T, Rasmussen JP, Howardy P, Mitchel J (1978) Respiratory thoraco-abdominal coordination and muscle fatigue in acute respiratory failure (Abstr.). Am Rev Respir Dis 117:89

Andersen JB, Kann T, Rasmussen JP, Qvist J (1979) Intermittent mandatory ventilation assists the diaphragm in weaning patients from mechanical ventilation. Dan Med Bull 26(7):363

Askanazi J, Rosenbaum SH, Hyman AI, Rosenbaum L, Milic-Emili J, Kinney JM (1980) Effects of parenteral nutrition on ventilatory drive. Anaesthesilogy 53(3):S185

Aubier M, Murciano D, Lecocguic Y, Viires N, Jacquens Y, Squara P, Pariente R (1985) Effect of hypophosphatemia on diaphragmatic contractility in patients with acute respiratory failure. New Eng J Med 313(7):420–424

Baratz RA, Philbin DM, Patterson RW (1971) Plasma antidiuretic hormone and urinary output during continuous positive-pressure breathing in dogs. Anaesthesiology 34(6):510–513

Benzer H (1982) The value of intermittent mandatory ventilation. Intensive Care Med 8(6):267–268

Bone RG, Francis PD, Pierce AK (1975) Pulmonary barotrauma complicating positive end-expiratory pressure. Am Rev Respir Dis 111:921–922

Boynton BR, Mannino FL, Davis RF, Kopotic RJ, Friederichsen G (1984) Combined high-frequency oscillatory ventilation and intermittent mandatory ventilation in critically ill neonates. J Pediatr 105(2):297–302

Boysen PG, Hasten RW, Heenan TJ, Downs JB (1979) Comparison of synchronized and non-synchronized intermittent mandatory ventilation (Abstr). Am Rev Respir Dis 119:96

Brach BB, Yin F, Timms R, Moser K (1976) Reduced inspiratory effort during intermittent mandatory ventilation with PEEP. Crit Care Med 4(3):142–143

Braun N (1984) Respiratory muscle dysfunction. Heart Lung 13(4):327–338

Brochard L, Harf A, Lorino H, Lemaire F (1989) Inspiratory pressure support prevents diaphragmatic fatigue during weaning from mechanical ventilation. Am Rev Respir Dis 139:513–521

Brochard L, Rua F, Lorino J, Lemaire F, Harf A (1988) Suppression of extrawork of breathing due to the endotracheal tube (ET). Intensive Care Med [Suppl 1] 14:261

Bursztein S, Taitelman U, de Myttenaere S, Michelson M, Dahan E, Gepstein R, Edelman D, Melamed Y (1978) Reduced oxygen consumption in catabolic state with mechanical ventilation. Crit Care Med 6(2):162–164

Bynum LJ, Wilson JE III, Pierce AK (1976) Comparison of spontaneous and positive-pressure breathing in supine normal subjects. J Appl Physiol 41(3):341–347

Chiang H, Pontoppidan H, Wilson RS, Browne DRG, Katz A (1973) Respiratory muscle discoordination following prolonged mechanical ventilation (Abstr). Annual Meeting of the American Society of Anesthesiologists, Oct 7–11, San Francisco, pp 211–212

Chin WDN, Cheung HW, Driedger AA, Cunningham DG, Sibbald WJ (1985) Assisted ventilation in patients with preexisting cardiopulmonary disease; the effect on systemic oxygen consumption, and tissue perfusion variables. Chest 88(4):503–511

Christopher KL, Neff TA, Bowman JL, Eberle DJ, Good JT (1985) Demand and continuous flow intermittent mandatory ventilation systems. Chest 87(5):625–630

Cohen CA, Zagelbaum G, Gross D, Roussos C, Macklem PT (1982) Clinical manifestations in inspiratory muscle fatigue. Am J Med 73:308–316

Colgan FJ, Barrow RE, Fanning GL (1971) Constant positive-pressure breathing and cardiorespiratory function. Anaesthesiology 34:145–151

Cournand A, Motley HL, Werko L, Richards DW (1948) Physiological studies of the effects of intermittent positive pressure breathing on cardiac output in man. Am J Physiol 152:162–174

Cullen P, Modell JH, Kirby RR, Klein EF, Long W (1975) Treatment of flail chest; use of intermittent mandatory ventilation and positive end-expiratory pressure. Arch Surg 110:1099–1103

Culpepper JA, Rinaldo JE, Rogers RM (1985) Effect of mechanical ventilator mode on tendency towards respiratory alkalosis. Am Rev Respir Dis 132:1075–1077

DeLemos RA, McLaughlin GW (1973) Techniques of ventilation in the newborn; the use of intermittent mandatory ventilation. Colloquium Sept 27–28, Pont-a-Mousson, pp 173–178

Downs JB, Klein EF Jr, Desautels D, Modell JH, Kirby RR (1973) Intermittent mandatory ventilation: a new approach to weaning patients from mechanical ventilators. Chest 64(3):331–335

Downs JB, Block AJ, Vennum KB (1974a) Intermittent mandatory ventilation in the treatmet of patients with chronic obstructive pulmonary disease. Anesth Analg 53(3):437–441

Downs JB, Perkins HM, Modell JH (1974b) Intermittent mandatory ventilation: an evaluation. Arch Surg 109:519–523

Downs JB, Douglas ME, Sanfelippo PM, Stanford W, Hodges MR, (1977) Ventilatory pattern, intrapleural pressure and cardiac output. Anaesth Analg 56(1):88–96

Fricker HS, Palla C, Mettler M (1980) Intermittierend obligate Beatmung in der Behandlung des idiopathischen Atemnotsyndroms bei Neugeborenen. Schweiz Med Wochenschr 110(7):251–255

Froese AB, Bryan AC (1974) Effects of anaesthesia on paralysis on diaphragmatic mechanics in man. Anaesthesiology 41(3):242–255

Gertz I, Hedenstierna G, Hellers G, Wahren J (1977) Muscle metabolism in patients with chronic obstructive lung disease and acute respiratory failure. Clin Sci Mol Med 52:395–403

Hastings PR, Bushnell LS, Skillman JJ, Weintraub RM, Hedley-Whyte J (1980) Cardiorespiratory dynamics during weaning with IMV versus ventilation in good-risk cardiac-surgery patients. Anaesthesiology 53(5):429–431

Heenan TJ, Downs JB, Douglas ME, Ruiz BC, Jumper L (1980) Intermittent mandatory ventilation; is synchronization important? Chest 77(5):598–602

Herrera M, Blasco J, Venegas J, Barba R, Doblas A, Marquez E (1985) Mouth occlusion pressure ($P_{0.1}$) in acute respiratory failure. Intensive Care Med 11:134–139

Herve P, Simonneau G, Girard P, Cerrina J, Mathieu M, Duroux P (1983) Total parenteral nutrition induces hypercapnia in mechanically ventilated patients with chronic respiratory insufficiency. Am Rev Respir Dis 127(4):255

Hewitt PB, Chamberlain JH, Seed RF (1973) The effect of carbon dioxide on cardiac output in patients undergoing mechanical ventilation following open heart surgery. Br J Anaesth 45:1035–1042

Hillman K, Friedloss J, Davey A (1986) A comparison of intermittent mandatory ventilation systems. Crit Care Med 14(5):499–502

Holle RHO, Montgomery AB, Schoene RB, Rindfleisch S, Pierson DJ, Hudson LD (1982) High central respiratory drives in patients who fail ventilator weaning. Am Rev Respir Dis 127 [Suppl] 2:88

Hooper RG, Browning M (1985) Acid-base changes and ventilator mode during maintenance ventilation. Crit Care Med 13(1):44–45

Hudson LD, Hurlow RS, Craig KC, Pierson DH (1985) Does intermittent mandatory ventilation correct respiratory alkalosis in patients receiving assisted mechanical ventilation? Am Rev Respir Dis 132:1071–1074

Jones JG (1977) The chest wall—tone and movement. Anaesthesiology 47(4):325–326

Jones JG (1987) Anaesthesia, and atelectasis; the role of V_{TAB} and the chest wall. Br J Anesth 59(8):949–953

Kanak R, Fahey PJ, Vanderwarf C (1985) Oxygen cost of breathing. Changes dependent upon mode of mechanical ventilation. Chest 87(1):126–127

Kety S, Schmidt CF (1946) The effects of active and passive hyperventilation on cerebral blood flow, cerebral oxygen consumption, cardiac output, and blood pressure in normal young men. J Clin Invest 25:107–119

Khambatta HJ, Baratz RA (1972) IPPB, plasma ADH, and urine flow in conscious man. J Appl Physiol 33:362–364

Khambatta HJ, Sullivan SF (1973) Effects of respiratory alkalosis on oxygen consumption and oxygenation. Anaesthesiology 38(1):53–58

Kirby R (1977) Intermittent mandatory ventilation in the neonate. Crit Care Med 5(1): 18–22

Kirby RR, Robison EJ, Schulz J, deLemos R (1971) A new pediatric volume ventilator. Anesth Analg 50(4):533–537

Kirby R, Robison E, Schulz J, deLemos RA (1972) Continuous-flow ventilation as an alternative to assisted or controlled ventilation in infants. Anaesth Analg 51(6):871–875

Kirby RS, Perry JC, Calderwood HW, Ruiz BC, Lederman DS, (1975) Cardiorespiratory effects of high positive end-expiratory pressure. Anaesthesiology 43(5):533–539

Kirby RF, Downs JB, Civetta JM, Modell JH, Dannemiller FJ, Klein EF, Hodges M (1981) High level positive end-expiratory pressure (PEEP) in acute respiratory insufficiency. Chest 67(2):156–163

Kumar A, Pontoppidan HH, Falke KJ, et al. (1973) Pulmonary barotrauma during mechanical ventilation. Crit Care Med 1:181

Kumar A, Pontoppidan H, Baratz RA, Laver MB (1974) Inappropriate response to increased plasma ADH during mechanical ventilation in acute respiratory failure. Anesthesiology 40(3):215–221

Laaban JP, Lemaire F, Baron JF, Trunet P, Harf A, Bonnet JL, Teisseire B (1985) Influence of caloric intake on the respiratory mode during mandatory minute volume ventilation. Chest 87(1):67–72

Luce JM, Pierson DJ, Hudson LD (1981) Intermittent mandatory ventilation. Chest 79(6):678–685

MacIntyre NR (1986) Respiratory function during pressure support ventilation. Chest 89(5):677–683

Marino W, Braun NMT (1982) Reversal of the clinical sequelae of respiratory muscle fatigue by intermittent mechanical ventilation (Abstr). Am Rev Respir Dis 125 (Pt 2):85

Mathru M, Rao TLK, El-Etr AA, Pifarre R (1982) Haemodynamic response to changes in ventilatory patterns in patients with normal and poor left ventricular reserve. Crit Care Med 10(7):423–426

Newman JH, Neff TA, Ziporin P (1977) Acute respiratory failure associated with hypophosphatemia. N Engl J Med 296(19):1101–1103

Nunn JF (1961) The distribution of inspired gas during thoracic surgery. Ann R Coll Surg Engl 28:223–237

Petersen GW, Baier H (1983) Incidence of pulmonary barotrauma in a medical ICU. Crit Care Med 11(2):67–69

Quan SF, Falltrick RT, Schlobohm RM (1981) Extubation from ambient or expiratory positive airway pressure in adults. Anesthesiology 55:53–56

Qvist J, Pontoppidan H, Wilson RS, Lowenstein E, Laver MB (1975) Haemodynamic responses to mechanical ventilation with PEEP: the effect of hypervolemia. Anaesthesiology 42(1):45–55

Rehder K, Sessler AD, Rodarte JE (1977) Regional intrapulmonary gas distribution in awake and anesthetized-paralysed man. J Appl Physiol 42(3):391–402

Rochester DF, Arora NS (1983) Respiratory muscle failure. Med Clin North Am 67(3):573–597

Rochester DF, Braun NMT, Laine S (1977) Diaphragmatic energy expenditure in chronic respiratory failure. Am J Med 63:223–232

Roussos C, Macklem PT (1982) The respiratory muscles. N Engl J Med 307(13):786–797

Samodelov LF, Falke KJ (1988) Total inspiratory work with modern demand valve devices compared to continuous flow CPAP. Intensive Care Med (in press) 14:632–639

Santak B, Raderacher P, Falke KJ (1988) Influence of SIMV on VA/Q distributions during postoperative weaning. Intensive Care Med [Suppl 1] 14:210

Schlobohm RM, Falltrick RT, Quan SF, Katz JA (1981) Lung volumes, oxygenation during spontaneous positive-pressure ventilation; the advantage of CPAP over EPAP. Anesthesiology 55:416–422

Shapiro BA, Cane RD (1984) The IMV–AMV controversy: a plea for clarification and redirection. Crit Care Med 12(5):472–473

Shutack JG, Fox WW, Shaffer TH, Schwartz JG (1982) Effect of low-rate intermittent mandatory ventilation on pulmonary function of low birth-weight infants. J Pediatr 100(5):799–802

Simonneau G, Lemaire F, Harf A, Carlet J, Teisseire B (1982) A comparative study of the cardiorespiratory effects of continuous positive airway pressure breathing and continuous positive pressure ventilation in acute respiratory failure. Intensive Care Med 8:61–67

Steinhoff H, Falke K, Schwarzhoff W (1982) Enhanced renal function associated with intermittent mandatory ventilation in acute respiratory failure. Intensive Care Med 8:69–74

Steinhoff HH, Kohlhoff RJ, Falke KJ (1984) Facilitation of renal function by intermittent mandatory ventilation. Intensive Care Med 10:59–65

Taylor RF, Marini JJ, Smith TC, Lamb VJ (1987) Bedside estimation of respiratory drive during machine assisted ventilation. Am Rev Respir Dis 135:A51

Tobin MJ, Perez W, Guenther SM, Semmes BJ, Mador MJ, Allen SJ, Lodato RF, Dantzker DR (1986) The pattern of breathing during successful and unsuccessful trials of weaning from mechanical ventilation. Am Rev Respir Dis 134(6):1111–1118

Trichet B, Falke K, Togut A, Laver MB (1975) The effect of pre-existing pulmonary vascular disease on the response to mechanical ventilation with PEEP following open-heart surgery. Anesthesiology 42(1):56–67

Venus B, Jacobs K, Mathru M (1980) Haemodynamic responses to different modes of mechanical ventilation in dogs with normal and acid aspirated lungs. Crit Care Med 8(11):620–627

Vuori A, Klossner J (1981) Central haemodynamics and oxygen transport during CPAP with and without mandatory ventilation. Acta Anaesthesiol Scand. 25:282–285

Vuori A, Jalonen J, Laaksonen V (1979) Continuous positive airways pressure during mechanical and spontaneous ventilation. Acta Anaesthesiol Scand 23:453–461

Watson WE, Smith AC, Spalding MB (1962) Transmural central venous pressure during intermittent positive pressure respiration. Br J Anaesth 34:278–286

Weisman IM, Rinaldo JE, Rogers RM, Sanders MH (1983) State of the art: intermittent mandatory ventilation. Am Rev Respir Dis 127:641–647

Wolff G, Brunner JX, Gradel E (1986) Gas exchange during mechanical ventilation and spontaneous breathing; intermittent mandatory ventilation after open heart surgery. Chest 90(1):11–17

Zarins CK, Bayne CG, Rice CL, Peters RM, Virgilio RW (1977) Does spontaneous ventilation with IMV protect from PEEP-induced cardiac output depression? J Surg Res 22(3):299–303

Continuous Positive Airway Pressure

A. Braschi and G. Iotti

Continuous positive airway pressure (CPAP) ventilation means spontaneous breathing with positive end expiratory pressure (PEEP). In this mode, ventilation depends upon the patient, while the machine serves only to maintain an airway pressure which is constantly higher than atmospheric pressure, and to control oxygen concentration, temperature, and humidity of the inspired gas.

In the adult acute respiratory distress syndrome (ARDS), the application of PEEP, together with controlled mechanical ventilation (CMV), has proved to be useful for the treatment of hypoxemia. Thus, CMV, originally developed for the treatment of pure ventilatory defects, such as poliomyelitis (Lassen 1953), was successfully employed in patients with diseases of the pulmonary parenchyma. However, considering that these patients retain, at least initially, their ventilatory potential, it was logical to propose a different approach, such as CPAP.

Gregory et al. (1971) first proposed CPAP in pediatrics, while Civetta et al. (1972) extended the application to adults. In any event, the idea was not completely new. Mention of its earlier use in both civil and military medicine can be found (Barach 1937; Barach et al. 1938, 1946; Bunnell 1912; Gagge et al. 1945). After the failure of extracorporeal membrane oxygenation (ECMO) in the treatment of ARDS (National Heart and Lung Institute 1974; Lemaire and Rapin 1980) demanded a reevaluation of simpler methods and has contributed to the further dissemination of CPAP. Presently CPAP is considered the method of choice in many types of acute respiratory failure of parenchymal origin. The low pressure levels used in CPAP make it the therapeutic technique closest to physiological breathing as well as the least barotraumatic.

The advantages and disadvantages of this technique will be outlined, but first we would like to point out that the main problem is clinical tolerance, which is partly determined by the technical characteristics of the apparatus.

CPAP Systems: Technical Notes

Optimal Characteristics

Before beginning an in-depth discussion of this topic, it would be worthwhile to analyze the differences that exist between natural spontaneous breathing (SB) and SB through a mechanical ventilator and associated equipment.

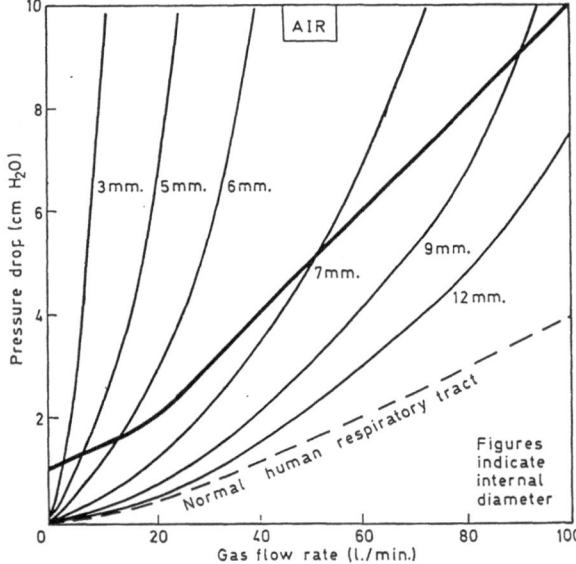

Fig. 1. Flow rate/pressure drop plots of a range of endotracheal tubes. *Heavy line* is the upper limit of acceptable resistance for an adult. (From Nunn, 1977)

The artificial airway represents the first important difference, that is, when CPAP is not performed with a face mask. If the patient has had a tracheostomy, the problem is not too great, since the tracheostomy cannula offers little resistance to air flow. In most cases, however, an oro- or nasotracheal tube is inserted, which can offer enough resistance to produce clinical problems (Nunn 1977) (Fig. 1).

The second fundamental difference lies in the environment from which the patient breathes. The atmosphere has a practically infinite volume at constant pressure and is not influenced in any way by our respiration. The patient placed on CPAP, however, is in communication with an environment greatly reduced in size, represented by the circuit of the ventilation system. Therefore, there is depressurization during the inspiratory phase and hyperpressurization during expiration. Various techniques have been employed to minimize these phenomena in an attempt to imitate atmospheric respiration as closely as possible. The ideal CPAP system therefore is one which maintains a constant pressure throughout the entire breathing cycle, which should be equal to the predetermined PEEP. Obviously, the greater the peak inspiratory and expiratory flow rates, the more difficult it is to achieve this ideal situation. A poor system results in wide swings in pressure. In comparison with the ideal CPAP, greater negative pleural pressure changes are needed to maintain the same inspiratory flow rates, resulting in increased inspiratory work.

There are therefore two main sources of respiratory work overload in patients on CPAP. One is the high resistance of the artificial airway and the other is the pressure instability of the circuit. Whenever the patient's strength becomes insufficient, this overload will be reflected in hypoventilation.

Demand Flow Systems

Demand flow is probably the most widely employed solution to the above-mentioned problems. It is based on the synergistic action of two valves, one for inspiration (demand valve) and one for expiration. As the patient attempts to inspire, the resulting circuit pressure drop (or in some cases the initial inspiratory flow) causes the demand valve to open and the expiratory valve to close. Once opened, the demand valve delivers a gas flow which adjusts itself to the patient's demands, although with a certain delay. The cycling from the inspiratory to the expiratory phase, i.e., closure of the demand valve and opening of the expiratory valve, comes about as a response to the expiratory demand of the patient. The signal consists of either a critical pressure increase in the respiratory circuit or a critical reduction of the inspiratory flow.

Demand flow is the technical solution usually employed by high performance ventilators which offer CPAP among various ventilation modes. Generally these machines do not use an additional valve to deliver the demand flow. When CPAP is selected, the inspiratory valve of the ventilator is made to function on demand. This enables the patient to condition both the timing and the degree of opening of the valve, i.e., the flow delivered.

A series of tests performed on various types of demand flow systems with an active lung simulator (Iotti et al. 1984) has shown that the initial phase of inspiration, and often expiration, is characterized by high resistance and zero or near-zero flow (Braschi et al. 1986b). Therefore, there is a delay in reaching the effective ventilation stage (Fig. 2). This latency varies from system to system and is inversely proportional to the force generated by the patient. This phenomenon probably has clinical relevance and may explain intolerance of some patients to CPAP and intermittent mechanical ventilation (IMV). The effect of these phases of high resistance and zero or near-zero flow (Iotti et al. 1985) is a reduction in effective ventilation time and therefore a potential reduction in tidal volume, especially if the patient is incapable of generating high transpulmonary pressures. On the other hand, with certain ventilators CPAP is poorly tolerated even by

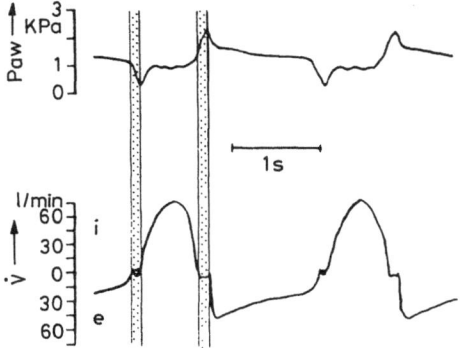

Fig. 2. CPAP through a demand flow system: shutter effect of valves. Airway pressure (Paw) and flow rate ($\dot{V}$) recording. High resistance phases can be seen at the beginning of inspiration (i) and expiration (e), with zero flow peaks in pressure. (From Iotti et al. 1985)

patients able to generate adequate transpulmonary pressures. This may be due to the shutter of the valves, which occurs twice during each respiratory cycle.

Among the various types of ventilators there are also marked differences in pressure levels during the effective ventilation phase. During inspiration there may be hypo-, normo-, or hyperpressurization. In the first case, the ventilator increases the respiratory work, in the second it remains neutral, and in the third it produces a mini-insufflation, like a low level pressure support ventilation. During expiration, the pressure level may be much higher than PEEP, due to an excessive resistance of the expiratory limb of the circuit, opposed to the patient's expiratory flow.

A number of studies dedicated to evaluation of CPAP systems are available in the literature (Braschi et al. 1986a, b; Cox et al. 1988; Falke and Samodelov 1986; Gibney et al. 1982; Katz et al. 1985; Samodelov and Falke 1988; Viale et al. 1985). The most commonly studied characteristic is inspiratory work. Katz in his thorough study (Katz et al. 1985) distinguishes between "additional work," which is the work the patient must add to overcome the ventilator, and "reduced work," which is the work performed by the machine on the respiratory system (Fig. 3). Using a different approach, the tidal volumes obtained with various systems were compared at constant inspiratory force (Braschi et al. 1986). Tidal volume was found to be low in those systems which hypopressurize during inspiration—i.e., added work—and high in those systems which hyperpressurize—i.e., reduced work.

However, a fair assessment cannot rest solely on the consideration of mechanical work. Though contributing to ventilation energy consumption, the

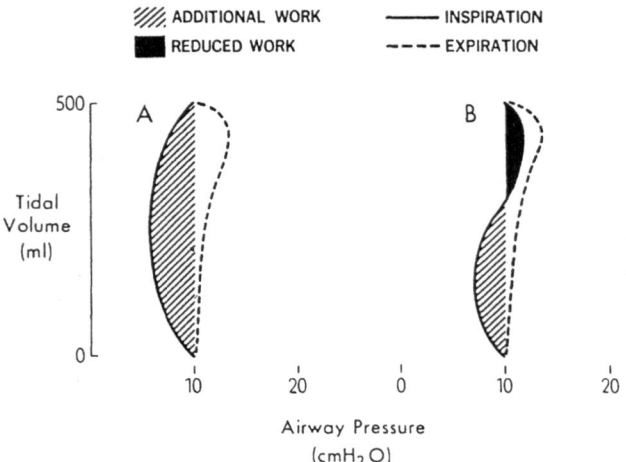

Fig. 3. Different kinds of pressure/volume loop during CPAP. (*A*) Airway pressure is below PEEP all along inspiration: this system demands an additional work of breathing of the patient. (*B*) After an initial drop, airway pressure exceeds PEEP, since inspiratory flow delivery is higher than demand: with this system some inspiratory work (reduced work) is performed by the ventilator. (From Katz et al. 1985)

high resistance phases cited above do not necessarily increase the mechanical work of breathing. They may only add an isovolumetric work (Falke and Samodelov 1986), which is not detectable on pressure-volume loops. We feel therefore that a complete evaluation of the subject must also include the duration of high resistance phases. This can explain, for instance, the remarkable difference between the Servoventilator 900 B and the Servoventilator 900 C: the first, poorly tolerated, is characterized by long delays, while the latter, much faster, has a good clinical performance.

In conclusion, the major problems in demand flow systems are their delay in valve opening and pressure instability. These problems have been reduced in the most recent machines and in the near future will probably be clinically irrelevant.

Continuous Flow Systems

Continuous flow systems are very simple, being a group of components placed in series through which a predetermined flow of fresh gas passes. The gas is delivered to the patient through a Y-piece and any excess gas is vented along with the patient's expired gas. A PEEP valve, placed at the end of the circuit, interacts with the gas flow to produce positive pressure. The various parts have been assembled in different ways, with the essential components being a gas supply which is adjustable for F_iO_2 and flow rate, a gas conditioner for heating and humidification, a manometer, and a PEEP device. The circuit should guarantee stable pressure and avoid the possibility of rebreathing. Thus, most continuous flow systems are equipped with a pressure stabilizer and one or more one-way valves.

As example of the numerous variations, we present diagrams of one of the most commonly used continuous flow systems (Fig. 4) and the one designed by Pelizzola et al. (1981) (Fig. 5), which we prefer. For a proper understanding of all these devices, it is first necessary to examine their individual components.

1. Gas supply. A mixer-flowmeter system can be used, or more simply a pair of flowmeters for air and O_2. An oximeter can be added for control of F_iO_2. The

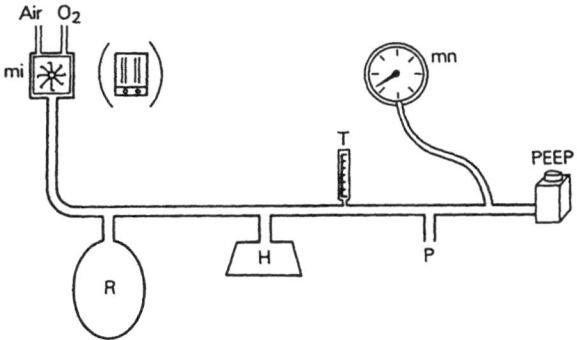

Fig. 4. Standard CPAP circuit. Air/O_2, gas supply; *mi*, mixer; *mn*, manometer; *R*, reservoir bag; *H*, heather-humidifer; *PEEP*, PEEP device; *T*, thermometer; *P*, patient

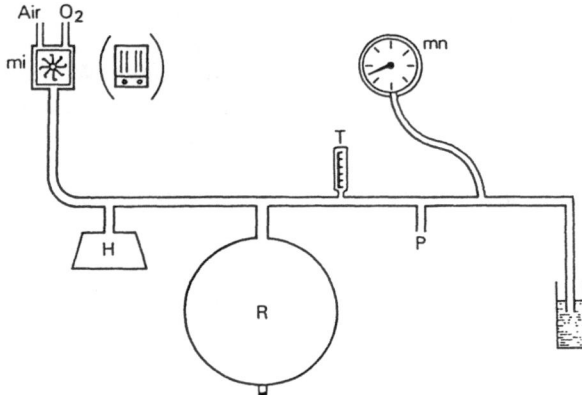

Fig. 5. CPAP circuit with high volume, high compliance reservoir bag. Legends as Fig. 4. Reservoir bag is a 10-l highly elastic latex balloon. PEEP device is an underwater seal

gas flow to be delivered depends on the patient's ventilation as well as on the circuit characteristics.

2. Gas conditioner. This must be a heater-humidifier able to handle high flow rates. If the gas conditioner is installed after the reservoir (see below and Fig. 4.4), it must offer low resistance to flow. If the device is not servocontrolled, a thermometer must be placed on the inspiratory limb near the Y-piece.

3. Manometer. This too should be placed in proximity to the patient and for safety should be equipped with high and low pressure alarms.

4. PEEP device. Without entering into the specific details of this component, which has been extensively described (Kacmarek et al. 1982a, b), it is useful to remember that a good PEEP valve should offer low resistance to flow so as not to cause excessive pressure increases during expiration or when the patient coughs. Furthermore, a flow-independent PEEP valve avoids the need to regulate the valve each time the fresh gas flow rate is modified (Hall et al. 1978). In spite of only fair performance, the most popular PEEP device remains the underwater seal, thanks to it simplicity and ease of use. Spring valves too are simple and convenient but not well suited to continuous flow systems (Braschi et al. 1985).

5. Pressure stabilizer. In a continuous flow circuit the simplest method of stabilizing pressure is to employ a fresh gas flow which exceeds the patient's peak inspiratory flow. This high flow rate, however, causes excessive gas waste, makes heating and humidification unreliable, and creates problems related to the PEEP device. Pressure stabilizers were therefore introduced to allow lower working flow rates. Civetta et al. (1972) proposed a reservoir made of a low compliance 5-l anesthesia balloon, but a stabilizer of this type performs inadequately and requires a fresh gas flow rate which is much higher than minute ventilation (Garg and Hill 1975; Gherini et al. 1979; Gibney et al. 1982). Various modifications were then proposed to improve the reservoir's performance. These include weight loading (Pfitzner 1976; Zebrowsky and Geer 1981), increased volume (Thomas et al. 1979), increased compliance (Ambu-CPAP), or an increase in both volume and compliance (Pelizzola et al. 1981).

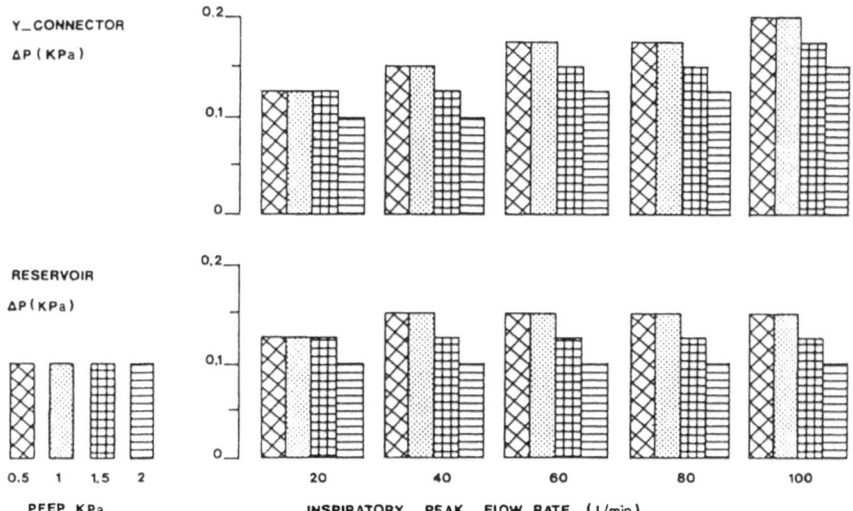

Fig. 6. CPAP circuit with high volume, high compliance reservoir bag (model evaluation): inspiratory pressure drop at the Y-piece and inside the reservoir, with different inspiratory peak flow rates (IPF) and different PEEP levels. Pressure drop is very low, not influenced by fresh gas flow rate, and reduced by increases of PEEP level. At the Y-piece the pressure drop is proportional to the IPF, while inside the reservoir it is not influenced by the IPF. (From Braschi et al. 1985)

The combination of increased volume and increased compliance offers excellent performance, i.e., stable pressure at low flow rates (Fig. 6). Here we will describe the characteristics of this type of system (Fig. 5) (Braschi et al. 1985). A highly elastic latex balloon is inserted in the circuit after the gas conditioner, near the Y-piece. The reservoir has a volume of approximately 10 l at atmospheric pressure and relatively constant compliance over a wide range of pressures. Compliance values are: $400 \, ml/cm \, H_2O$ at 5–10 cm H_2O, $500 \, ml/cm \, H_2O$ at 15 cm H_2O, and $700 \, ml/cm \, H_2O$ at 20 cm H_2O. At higher pressure, there is danger of rupture of the balloon. The secret of this reservoir lies in its elevated compliance which remains constant over a wide range of volumes. When the circuit is pressurized, it can release a tidal volume without any significant change in the compliance of the reservoir. Since this compliance is very high, the volume reduction will be followed by just a minimal pressure decrease (Fig. 6). Moreover, since the reservoir is recharged during the initial phase of expiration, it also acts to amplify flow. The flow rate offered to the patient at the beginning of inspiration is always higher than the flow rate from the gas source (Fig. 7). For maximal efficiency of the pressure stabilizer, the resistance of the circuit between the reservoir and the patient must be minimal. For this reason, the reservoir should be placed near the Y-piece and neither the humidifier nor a one-way valve should be inserted between the two (Fig. 6).

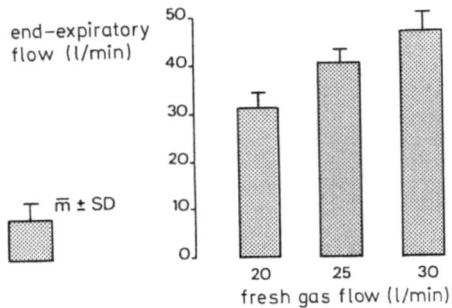

Fig. 7. CPAP circuit with high volume high compliance reservoir bag (model evaluation): end-expiratory continuous flow through the Y-piece with different fresh gas flow rates. Flow rate offered to the patient at the start of inspiration is always 60% higher than flow rate from the gas source. (Data from Braschi et al. 1985)

6. One-way valves. A one-way valve in the expiratory limb is necessary to avoid rebreathing from this side of the circuit. The PEEP valve is commonly used for this purpose. Besides that, there may be the danger of a certain amount of retrograde expiration towards the reservoir, with subsequent rebreathing. In the absence of one-way valves on the inspiratory limb of the circuit, retrograde expiration depends on the balance between the patient's expiratory flow, flow from the gas source, volume and compliance of the reservoir, and resistance to expiration determined mainly by the PEEP device. When a circuit has an inefficient pressure stabilizer, the high gas flow necessary to maintain a stable pressure opposes retrograde expiration, forming a sort of pneumatic valve. The problem becomes real, however, when the high volume, high compliance latex reservoir is used, due to the low flow rates which can be employed and to the high compliance which permits easy entry of expired gas into the reservoir itself. There are two solutions to the problem:

1. Maintaining gas flow rate above 30 l/min with a low resistance PEEP device, such as an underwater seal. In this way, a convenient pneumatic valve able to handle almost all clinical situations is formed.
2. Insertion of a one-way valve between reservoir and Y-piece. Although the added inspiratory resistance may produce a slight fall in the performance of the system, the overall performance is excellent (Braschi et al. 1987).

In summary, when compared with demand flow systems, continuous flow systems maintain some important advantages such as: low cost, simplicity and, functionally, the absence of high resistance phases. In fact the continuous flow system is always ready to deliver inspiratory flows or receive expiratory flows, without any delay. The pressure stability can be very good (Braschi et al. 1985). The best performance is obtained using a high volume, high compliance reservoir and a circuit as indicated in Fig. 5, which, among other things, allows a relatively low working flow rate (30 l/min).

Mixed Systems

Some new ventilators can provide CPAP by means of mixed systems, working with a continuous flow (base flow) that is increased on patient demand. The classical continuous flow system function is thus mimicked by ventilator servo-controlled valves, theoretically maintaining the advantages and removing the drawbacks of both continuous and demand flow technique.

Among these systems, the more original is the "Flow-by" system, provided as an optional function by the ventilator Puritan Bennett 7200a (Cox et al. 1988). A continuous flow between 5 and 20 l/min can be selected. Patient activity is monitored by continuous comparison of the flow rate delivered by the inspiratory valves and the flow rates passing through the expiratory port, thus collecting: (a) signals for modulation of the base flow, which is increased by the servocontrol system during inspiration, to match the patient's demand, and is decreased during expiration; (b) measurements of tidal and minute ventilation.

Problems in Monitoring

Demand flow systems are generally equipped with the standard ventilation monitors and alarms, usually concerning pressure, ventilation volumes F_iO_2, and sometimes capnometry. Thanks to these monitors, demand flow systems are safe even though their mechanical performance is not always satisfactory. The same control level in continuous flow systems would require a flow transducer placed at the junction between the circuit and the patient, outside of the continuous stream. Since the instrument is costly, hard to find, and is exposed to humidity and secretions which compromise its performance, it is not widely used.

Capnometry represents a good compromise for the monitoring of continuous flow systems. In addition to monitoring $ETCO_2$, a capnometer with alarms will signal apnea, disconnection, abnormal respiratory rates, and high inspiratory CO_2 concentrations due to rebreathing. This monitoring level can be defined as safe, but other systems can be added, such as the recent and interesting continuous noninvasive SaO_2 monitoring (Pulse Oximetry) (Harris 1987).

Physiologic Effects of CPAP

Respiratory effects

Volume Effect. This is the most important effect, due to the action of PEEP on the lungs. PEEP determines an increase in end-expiratory transpulmonary pressure, which gives an increase in end-expiratory lung volume or functional residual capacity (FRC) It is still not clear whether the increase in FRC obtained with CPAP is equal or superior to that obtained with the same level of expiratory positive airway pressure (EPAP). The latter consists of spontaneous ventilation with positive pressure during expiration and atmospheric pressure during inspiration (Gattinoni et al. 1980; Layon et al. 1986; Schlobohm et al. 1981). In any case the problem is academic, since CPAP is preferable because it imposes a lower work of breathing. It is of interest, however, to note the recent demonstration that at equal PEEP levels the increase in FRC is greater in CPAP

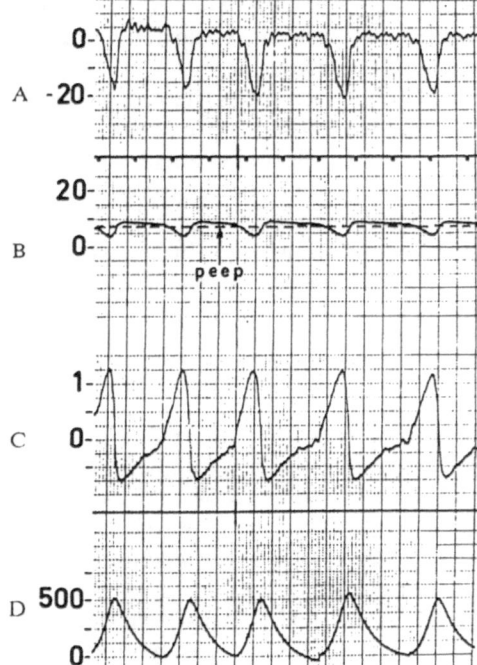

Fig. 8. CPAP circuit with high volume, high compliance reservoir bag. Recording of esophageal pressure (A_1 cm H_2O), airway pressure (B_1 cm H_2O), flow rate (C_1 l/s), and spirogram (D_1 ml). Good airway pressure stability, in spite of high values of minute ventilation and inspiratory peak flow rate

than in CMV-PEEP with paralysis (Mascheroni et al. 1986). The improvement in gas exchange depends on the volume effect which allows a recruitment of functionally excluded alveoli and/or a greater expansion of poorly functioning alveoli. Furthermore, the increase in FRC is accompanied by an improvement in static compliance as well be a reduction in airway resistance. Thus, both the elastic and frictional components of work of breathing are reduced (Katz and Marks 1985).

Pressure Effect. In any mode of ventilation, PEEP causes an elevation in both pleural and airway baseline pressures, due to hyperinflation of the respiratory system. The fundamental difference between CMV-PEEP and CPAP lies in the inspiratory phase. In the former, inspiration takes place thanks to hyperpressurization of the airways, which is accompanied by a further increase in pleural pressure, while in the latter the inspiratory muscles are used to create pleural depressurization. Thus, in CPAP, mean pleural pressure is lower than in CMV-PEEP. On the other hand, if we consider airway pressure, in CMV-PEEP there is a large inspiratory positive pressure wave, with a rapid expiratory return to near-PEEP levels. In CPAP, there is only a modest oscillation near baseline levels (Fig. 8), with a slight drop in inspiration, a slight increase during expiration, and mean pressure near PEEP. The fact that CPAP causes fewer hemodynamic repercussions at equal PEEP levels is explained by these lower pleural and alveolar pressures. The heart is less compressed causing less decrease of preload, and intraalveolar vessels are less compressed causing a lower increase in resistance.

Gas Exchange. CPAP improves arterial oxygenation through various mechanisms, the most important of which is the reopening of collapsed alveoli and the consequent reequilibration of the ventilation/perfusion ratios and reduction in venous admixture. Furthermore, there is better distribution of inspired gas and better capillary perfusion and improved cardiac output with an occasional increase in $P\bar{v}O_2$. In this way there is a net increase in O_2 delivery (Fig. 9).

The problem of CO_2 elimination during CPAP is more complex. There is often a tendency toward hypercapina. It is of primary importance to check if this is due to rebreathing (see above). In the absence of rebreathing, the CO_2 increase is usually due to increased work of breathing or to overdistension of the alveoli with increased dead space. This phenomenon may also occur during CMV-PEEP, but with less clinical relevance due to lower CO_2 production caused by the absence of inspiratory work and sedation. However, hypercapina during CPAP, as long as $PaCO_2$ remains under 50 mmHg, is of less concern than during

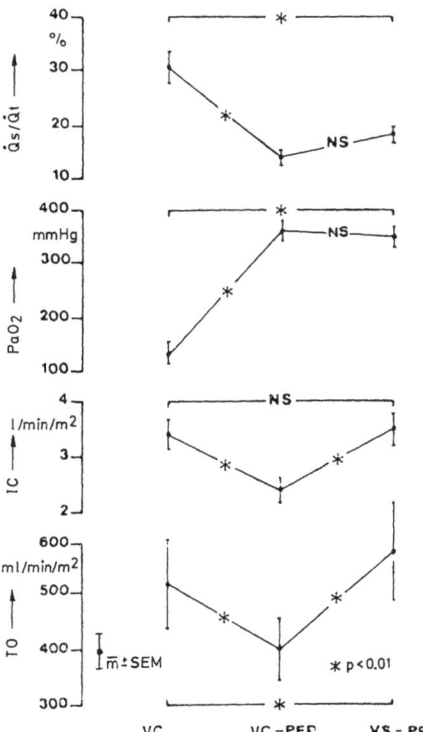

Fig. 9. Intrapulmonary shunt ($\dot{Q}s/\dot{Q}t$), PaO_2, cardiac index (IC), and oxygen delivery (TO_2) during CMV (VC), CMV-PEEP (VC-PEP), and CPAP (VS-PEP). Best oxygen delivery is observed with CPAP, since cardiac index is maintained while PaO_2 is increased. (Data from Simonneau et al. 1982)

spontaneous breathing without PEEP, in which it reflects alveolar hypoventilation and is accompanied by hypoxemia. Alveolar hypoventilation rarely causes hypoxemia during CPAP because of the volume effect on the alveoli and control of F_iO_2.

Hemodynamic Effects

Any increase in intrathoracic pressure causes decreased cardiac performance (Cournand et al. 1946). This becomes particularly relevant in the presence of continuous, high pressure increases such as in CMV with high PEEP levels. At equal PEEP levels, CPAP provides better hemodynamic tolerance compared with CMV-PEEP. The change from spontaneous ventilation in ambient air to CPAP either does not modify cardiac output (Downs et al. 1977; Sturgeon et al. 1977) or causes a slight reduction (Marquez et al. 1979; Perschau et al. 1979; Schlemmer et al. 1981; Vuori 1980) proportional to the PEEP level employed (Vuori 1980). On the other hand, the same PEEP level with CMV causes greater hemodynamic interference (Marquez et al. 1979; Simonneau et al. 1982; Vuori et al. 1979). The effects of CPAP therefore appear identical or less significant than those of CMV without PEEP (Fig. 9) (Downs et al. 1977; Simonneau et al. 1982).

The reduction in cardiac output observed during CPAP is due to a decrease in left ventricular stroke volume (Jardin et al. 1981; Marquez et al. 1979; Perschau et al. 1979; Schlemmer et al. 1981; Vuori 1980). This is related to a reduction in preload, with decreased filling pressure (Marquez et al. 1979; Perschau et al. 1979) and end-diastolic volume (Jardin et al. 1984; Schlemmer et al. 1981). It seems that the alterations of the left ventricle are mainly due to the effect of increased intrathoracic pressure on the right heart. In fact PEEP application causes an immediate reduction in the right ventricular stroke volume, while the left ventricular stroke volume drops more slowly (Perschau et al. 1979).

These observations and the finding of right ventricle dilatation (Jardin et al. 1984) suggest the possibility of direct action of increased pulmonary vascular resistance on the right ventricle. The repercussions on the left ventricle would therefore seem indirect (Jardin et al. 1984) and secondary to the reduction in right ventricle stroke volume with diminished pulmonary venous return (Perschau et al. 1979). It should be noted, however, that all the studies in which hemodynamic interference due to CPAP was demonstrated, were performed on subjects who were healthy or at least had no pulmonary disease. It is possible that in ARDS patients CPAP improves both respiratory and hemodynamic conditions (Dhainaut et al. 1987).

Finally, concerning the different CPAP methods, the use of systems with low capacity of pressurization and high inspiration-expiration gradients does not seem to offer substantial hemodynamic advantages (Weinstein et al. 1978). Furthermore, no significant differences were observed between demand flow and continuous flow systems (Vuori 1981), so the type of system can be chosen independently of hemodynamic considerations.

Effect on Extrathoracic Organs

Mechanical ventilation with PEEP has a series of secondary effects on the main extrathoracic organs (Suter 1981). The renal effects are the best known and consist of sodium and water retention accompanied by increased plasma or urinary ADH levels (Berry 1981). The renal effects of CPAP have been compared with those observed during controlled ventilation, and the adverse effects on renal function are fewer with CPAP (Hemmer et al. 1980). We are not aware of analogous studies to the effects on other organs, but it is reasonable to assume that the more favorable hemodynamic conditions obtained during CPAP tend to improve the function of other organs and systems, particularly the liver and central nervous system.

Indications

The main indication for CPAP is acute respiratory failure with hypoxemia when spontaneous ventilation is efficient, especially when hypoxemia is due to pulmonary edema both cardiogenic or noncardiogenic. CPAP presently represents the first line of treatment in the initial forms of ARDS. Gattinoni et al. (1984) have noted that a static respiratory system compliance of less than 30 ml/cm H_2O, as in advanced severe ARDS, usually predicts failure of CPAP. Poor tolerance can be defined by $PaCO_2$ greater than 50 mmHg, respiratory rate greater than 40/min, tidal volume lower than 300 ml, hemodynamic alterations, and clinical signs like agitation and sweating.

Thoracic trauma is another indication, even in the presence of extensive lesions of the chest wall. The classical orthopaedic concept of internal pneumatic stabilization of the flail chest is outdated. More realistically, the problem lies in the underlying pulmonary parenchyma. Pulmonary edema in the area of the contusion reduces compliance and requires excessive inspiratory pleural negative pressures, with deleterious effects on the flail chest. CPAP can help to overcome the critical phase relatively quickly, indeed often more quickly than with classical ventilation (Dittman et al. 1982). Intubation can sometime be avoided in these patients, thereby reducing the risk of superimposed respiratory infections When CPAP is performed through a face mask, however, gastric distension may occur, which can be particularly dangerous in surgical patients. There have also been cases of pneumoencephalus in patients with fractures of the base of the skull (Klopfenstein et al. 1980).

The prophylactic value of CPAP or CMV-PEEP in patients at risk for ARDS is still an open question (Shapiro et al. 1984). Presently there are no clinical or experimental data which unequivocally demonstrate the prophylactic efficacy of PEEP in the prevention of ARDS. Some clinical studies (Schmidt et al. 1976; Valdes et al. 1978; Wergelt et al. 1979) have found positive results in this regard, but they must be interpreted with caution due to the difficulties in defining "patients at risk" and to the lack of uniform diagnostic criteria for ARDS.

Atelectasis. Diffuse microatelectasis and basal atelectasis are frequently encountered in the postoperative period. Some authors have found PEEP (Fowler et al. 1978) and especially CPAP (Andersen et al. 1980; Covelli et al. 1982; Williamson and Modell 1982) to be useful in the treatment of atelectasis. Andersen et al. (1979) designed an experimental model and showed that one mechanism of the FRC increase by CPAP is an increase of collateral ventilation to collapsed alveoli, a concept now confirmed by other studies (Anderes et al. 1979; Carlsson et al. 1981).

Weaning from CMV. Whenever a prolonged period of CMV-PEEP is necessary for treatment of a severe form of respiratory failure, the patient must be retrained to perform respiratory work and spontaneous ventilation. CPAP, sometimes following a period of IMV-PEEP (Feeley et al. 1975), is useful for this purpose. The weaning process should consist of a progressive reduction in PEEP and FiO_2. It is also important to remember that an endotracheal tube suppresses the function of the glottis, hence reducing FRC and pulmonary compliance, and increasing respiratory work. Thus spontaneous ventilation with a tracheal tube in place and without PEEP can create problems (Annest et al. 1980; Quan et al. 1981). Furthermore, in this situation efficient expectoration is impossible and clearance of secretions from the respiratory tree is reduced. CPAP, even with low PEEP levels, substitutes for the glottis in maintaining a positive airway pressure, thereby preventing microatelectasis.

Uncommon Indications. Finally, we would like to cite some of the unique indications reported in the literature. The treatment of asthma attacks (Martin et al. 1982; Tenaillon et al. 1983) with CPAP merits further evaluation; its rationale is actually very attractive (Marini 1989). In pediatrics CPAP has been useful in the treatment of severe forms of tracheobronchomalacia (Kanter et al. 1982) and unilateral diaphragmatic paralysis (Robotham et al. 1980). Nasal CPAP has been used for management of obstructive sleep apnea (Sullivan et al. 1981), and face mask CPAP has been successfully employed for treatment of left ventricular failure complicated by respiratory insufficiency in acute myocardial infarction (Räsänen et al. 1985). Correctly titrated CPAP is an efficient way of reducing the work of breathing due to auto-PEEP (Petrof et al. 1990).

Conclusion

The major advantages of CPAP with respect to other mechanical ventilation techniques have been discussed. In summary they are: (a) the CPAP method is very close to spontaneous ventilation; (b) its pulmonary, hemodynamic, and extrathoracic side effects are much more limited than those of CMV-PEEP; (c) it can be performed without intubation, with a simple face mask; (d) home-made equipment can be used, keeping costs very low.

   The limitations of CPAP, aside from the technical problems dicussed above, lie in the fact that it can only be used in patients with effective spontaneous ventilation. Adequate mental status and patient cooperation are necessary only when CPAP is performed with a face mask. Clinical tolerance must be evaluated very carefully. The absolute contraindications for CPAP are the same as those for PEEP, keeping in mind, however, that at a given PEEP level the mean intrathoracic pressure is much lower than during CMV-PEEP.

References

Anderes C, Anderes H, Gasser D (1979) Postoperative spontaneous breathing with CPAP to normalize late postoperative oxygenation. Intensive Care Med 5:15–21

Andersen JB, Qvist J, Kann T (1979) Recruiting collapsed lung through collateral channels with positive end-expiratory pressure. Scand J Respir Dis 60:260–266

Andersen JB, Olesen KP, Eikard E, Jansen E, Qvist J (1980) Periodic continuous positive airway pressure (CPAP) by mask in the treatment of atelectasis. Eur J Respir Dis 61:20–25

Annest S, Gottlieb M, Poloski WH (1980) Detrimental effects of removing end expiratory pressure prior to endotracheal extubation. Ann Surg 191:539–545

Barach AL (1937) Recent advances in inhalation therapy in the treatment of cardiac and respiratory disease. NT State J Med 37:1095–1110

Barach AL, Martin J, Eckman M (1938) Positive pressure respiration and its application to the treatment of acute pulmonary edema. Ann Intern Med 12:754–795

Barach AL, Eckman M, Ginsburg E (1946) Studies on positive pressure respiration I. General aspects and types of pressure breathing II. Effect on respiration and circulation at sea level. J Aviat med 17:290–320

Berry AJ (1981) Respiratory support and renal function. Anesthesiology 55:655–667

Braschi A, Iotti G, Locatelli A, Bellinzona G (1985) Functional evaluation of a CPAP circuit with high compliance reservoir bag. Intensive Care Med 11:85–89

Braschi A, Iotti G, Locatelli A, Bellinzona G, Bianchi T, Bobbio Pallavicini F (1986a) Différents systèmes pour VS-PEP: répercussions sur le volume courant. Reanim Soins Intensifs Med Urgence 2:263

Braschi A, Iotti G, Lacatelli A, Semenza GM, Bellinzona G, Cremaschi R, Bobbio Pallavicini F (1986b) High resistance phases in spontaneous breathing during mechanical ventilation (Abstr). Intensive Care Med 12:227

Braschi A, Iotti G, Lacatelli A, Bellinzona G, (1987) A continuous flow intermittent mandatory ventilation with continuous positive airway pressure with high-compliance reservoir bag. Crit Care Med 15:947–950

Bunnel S (1972) The use of nitrous oxide and oxygen to maintain anesthesia and positive pressure for thoracic surgery. JAMA 58:835–838

Carlsson C, Sonden B, Thylen U (1981) Can postoperative continuous positive airway pressure (CPAP) prevent pulmonary complications after abdominal surgery? Intensive Care Med 7:225–229

Civetta GM, Brons R, Gabel JD (1972) A simple and effective method of employing spontaneous positive pressure ventilation. J Thorac Cardiovasc Surg 63:312–317

Cournand A, Motley HL, Werko L, Richard DWJr (1948) Physiological studies of the effects of intermittent positive pressure breathing on cardiac output in man. Am J Physiol 152:162–174

Covelli HD, Weled BJ, Beckman JF (1982) Efficacy of continuous positive airway pressure administered by face mask. Chest 81:147–150

Cox D, Tinloi SF, Farrimond JG (1988) Investigation of the spontaneous mode of breathing of different ventilators. Intensive Care Med 14:532–537

Dhainaut JF, Aouate P, Monsallier JF, Devaux JY, Brunet F, Huyghebaert MF, Villmant D, Armaganidis A, de Gournay JM (1987) Improvement of right ventricular performance by continuous positive airway pressure in adult respiratory distress syndrome. J Crit Care 2:15–21

Dittman M, Steenblock U, Krazlin M, Wolff G (1982) Epidural analgesia or mechanical ventilation for multiple rib fractures. Intensive Care Med 8:89–92

Downs JB, Douglas ME, Sanfelippo PM, Stanford W, Hodges MR (1977) Ventilatory pattern, intrapleural pressure, and cardiac output. Anesth Analg 56:88–94

Falke KJ, Samodelov LF (1986) Inspiratory work of breathing with CPAP systems. In: Vincent JL (ed) Update in intensive care and emergency medicine. Springer, Berlin Heidelberg New York, pp 96–100

Feeley TV, Saumarez R, Klick JM, McNabb TJ, Skillman JJ (1975) Positive end-expiratory pressure in weaning patients from controlled ventilation. A prospective randomized trial. Lancet 2:725–729

Fowler AA III, Scoggins WG, O'Donohue WJ Jr (1978) Positive end-expiratory pressure in the management of lobar atelectasis. Chest 74:497–500

Gagge AP, Allen SC, Marbarger AC (1945) Pressure breathing. J Aviat Med 16:2–8

Garg GP, Hill GE (1975) The use of spontaneous positive airway pressure (CPAP) for reduction of intrapulmonary shunting in adults with acute respiratory failure. Can Anaesth Soc. J 22:284–290

Gattinoni L, Pelizzola A, Rossi GP, Speciani A (1980) Functional residual capacity during end positive (EPAP) and continuous positive (CPAP) airway pressure in spontaneous breathing healthy subjects (Abstr). Intensive Care Med 6:47

Gattinoni L, Pesenti A, Caspani ML, Pellizzola A, Mascheroni D, Marcolin R, Iapichino G, Langer M, Agostini A, Kolobow T, Melrose DG, Damia G (1984) The role of total static lung compliance in the management of severe ARDS unresponsive to conventional treatment. Intensive Care Med 10:121–126

Gherini S, Peters RM, Virgilio RW (1979) Mechanical work of the lungs and work of breathing with positive end-expiratory pressure and continuous positive airway pressure. Chest 76:251–256

Gibney NRT, Wilson RS, Pontoppidan H (1982) Comparison of work of breathing on high gas flow and demand valve continuous positive airway pressure systems. Chest 82:692–695

Gregory GA, Kitterman JA, Phibbes RH, Tooley WH, Hamilton WK (1971) Treatment of ARDS with continuous positive airway pressure. N Engl J Med 284:1333–1340

Hall JR, Rendleman DC, Downs JB (1978) PEEP devices; flow dependent increases in airway pressure (Abstr). Crit Care Med 6:100

Harris K (1987) Noninvasive monitoring of gas exchange. Respir Care 32:544–553

Hemmer M, Viquerat CE, Suter PM, Vallotton MB (1980) Urinary antidiuretic hormone excretion during mechanical ventilation and weaning in man. Anaesthesiology 52:395–400

Iotti G, Braschi A, Locatelli A, Bellinzona G (1985) Respiration spontanée au cours de la ventilation artificielle: importance de la résistance des valves. Presse Med 14:165

Jardin F, Farcot JC, Boisante L, Curien N, Margairaz A, Bourdarias JP (1981) Influence of positive end-expiratory pressure on left ventricular performance. N. Engl. J. Med 304:387–392

Kacmarek RM, Dimas S, Reynolds J, Shapiro BA (1982a) Technical aspects of positive end-expiratory pressure (PEEP). I. Physics of PEEP devices. Respir Care 27:1478–1489

Kacmarek RM, Dimas S, Reynolds J, Shapiro BA (1982b) Technical aspects of positive end-expiratory pressure (PEEP). III. PEEP with spontaneous ventilation. Respir Care 27:1505–1518

Kanter RK, Pollack MM, Wright WW, Grunfast KM (1982) Treatment of severe tracheobronchomalacia with continuous positive airway pressure (CPAP) Anesthesiology 57:54–56

Katz JA, Marks JD (1985) Inspiratory work with and without continuous positive airway pressure in patients with acute respiratory failure. Anesthesiology 63:598–607

Katz JA, Kraemer RW, Gierde GE (1985) Inspiratory work and airway pressure with continuous positive airway pressure delivery systems. Chest 88:519–526

Klopfenstein CE, Forster A, Suter PM (1980) Pneumocephalus. A complication of continuous positive airway pressure after trauma. Chest 78:656–657

Lassen HCA (1983) A preliminary report on the 1952 epidemic of poliomyelitis in Copenhagen with special reference to the treatment of acute respiratory insufficiency. Lancet 37:41

Layon J, Banner MJ, Peterson CV, Gallaghert J, Modell JH (1986) Continuous positive airway pressure and expiratory positive airway pressure increase functional residual capacity equivalently. Chest 89:517–521

Lemaire F, Rapin M (1980) Des poumons artificiels dans l'insuffisance respiratoire aigue: un echec? Nouv Presse Med 9:3677–3679

Marini JJ (1989) Should PEEP be used in airflow obstruction? Am Rev Respir Dis 140:1–3

Marquez JM, Douglas ME, Downs JB, Wu WH, Mantini EL, Kuck EJ, Calderwood HW (1979) Renal function and cardiovascular responses during positive airway pressure. Anesthesiology 50:393–398

Martin JC, Shore S, Engel LA (1982) Effect of continuous positive airway pressure on respiratory mechanics and pattern of breathing in induced asthma. Am Rev Respir Dis 126:812–817

Mascheroni D, Langer M, Marcolin M, Ronzoni G, Fumagalli R, Gattinoni L (1986) Functional residual capacity is higher in CPAP than in CPPV with anaesthesia and on paralysis. Intensive Care Med 12:228

National Heart and Lung Institute (1974) Protocol for extracorporeal support of respiratory insufficiency, collaborative program. NIH, Bethseda

Nunn JF (1977) Resistance to gas flow. Applied respiratory physiology Butterworth London

Pelizzola A, Mascheroni D, Marcolin R, Prato P, Pesenti A, Gattinoni L, Damia G (1978) Reservoir ad alta compliance per l'ottimizzazione di un circuito di CPAP. Anest Rianim 22:279–288

Perschau RA, Pepine CJ, Nichols WW, Downs JB (1979) Instantaneous blood flow responses to positive end-expiratory pressure with spontaneous ventilation. Circulation 59:1312–1318

Petrof JP, Legaré M, Goldberg P, Milic-Emili J, Gottfried S (1990) CPAP reduces work of breathing and dysprea during weaning from mechanical ventilation in severe COPD. Am Rev Resp Dis 141:281–289

Pfitzner J (1976) Continuous positive airway pressure, the collection of expired gases. Anaesthesia 31:410–415

Quan SF, Falltick RT, Schlobohm RM (1981) Extubation from ambient or expiratory positive airway pressure in adults. Anesthesiology 55:53–56

Räsänen J, Vaisanen IT, Hikkila J, Nikki P (1985) Acute myocardial infarction complicated by left ventricular dysfunction and respiratory failure: the effects of continuous airway pressure. Chest 87:158–162

Robotham JL, Chipps BE, Shermeta DW (1980) Continuous positive airway pressure in hemidiaphragmatic paralysis. Anesthesiology 52:167–170

Samodelov LF, Falke KJ (1988) Total inspiratory work with modern demand valve devices compared to continuous flow CPAP. Intensive Care Med 14:632–639

Schlemmer B, de Vernejoul F, Dhainaut JF, Bons J, Weber S, Neveux E, Monsallier JF (1981) Effets de la ventilation spontanee en pression positive permanente (CPAP) sur la fonction ventriculaire gauche. Anesth Analg Reanim 38:537–540

Schlobohm RM, Falltrick RT, Quan SF, Katz JA (1981) Lung volumes, mechanics and oxygenation during spontaneous positive pressure ventilation: the advantage of CPAP over EPAP. Anesthesiology 55:416–422

Schmidt GB, O'Neill WW, Kotb K, Hwang KK, Bennet EJ, Bombeck CT (1976) Continuous positive airway pressure in the prophylaxis of the adult respiratory distress syndrome. Surg. Gynecol. Obstet 143:613–618

Shapiro BA, Cane RD, Harrison RA (1984) Positive end-expiratory pressure therapy in adults with special reference to acute lung injury: a review of the literature and suggested clinical correlation. Crit Care Med 12:127–141

Simonneau G, Lemaire F, Harf A, Carlet J, Teisseire B (1982) A comparative study of the cardiorespiratory effects of continuous positive airway pressure breathing and continuous positive pressure ventilation in acute respiratory failure. Intensive Care Med 8:61–67

Sturgeon CL, Douglas ME, Downs JB, Dannemiller FJ (1977) PEEP and CPAP: cardiopulmonary effects during spontaneous ventilation. Anesth Analg. 56:633–639

Sullivan CE, Issa FG, Berthon Jones M, Eves L (1981) Reversal of obstructive sleep apnea by continuous positive airway pressure through the nares. Lancet 1:862–865

Suter PM (1981) Les effets secondaires de la ventilation mécanique sur d'autres organes et systèmes. Ann Anesthesiol Fr 5:483–486

Tenaillon A, Salmona JP, Burdin M, Lissac J (1983) Continuous positive airway pressure in asthma. Am Rev Respir Dis 127:658

Thomas L, Robert D, Malquarti V, Gerard M, Kirkorian G, Bertoye A (1979) Travail respiratoire lors de la ventilation spontanée en pression positive continue: importance de la capacitance du circuit. Nouv Presse Med 8:45

Valdes ME, Powers SR, Sham DM, Newell JC, Scavill WA, Dutton RE (1978) Continuous positive airway pressure in prophylaxis of adult respiratory distress syndrome in trauma patients. Surg. Forum 29:187–189

Viale JP, Annat G, Bertrand O, Godard J, Motin J (1985) Additional inspiratory work in intubated patients breathing with continuous positive airway pressure systems. Anesthesiology 63:536–539

Vuori A, Effects of the level of CPAP on central haemodynamics and oxygen transport. Acta Anaesthesiol Scand 24:295–298

Vuori A (1981) Central haemodynamics, oxygen transport and oxygen consumption during three methods for CPAP. Acta Anaesthesiol Scand 25:376–380

Vuori A, Jalonen J, Laaksonen V (1979) Continuous positive airway pressure during mechanical and spontaneous ventilation. Acta Anaesthesiol Scand 23:453–461

Weinstein ME, Rice CL, Peters RM, Virgilio RW (1978) Hemodynamic and respiratory responses to varying gradients between end-expiratory pressure and end-inspiratory pressure in patients breathing on continuous positive airway pressure. J Trauma 18:231–235

Wergelt JA, Mitchell RA, Snyder WH (1979) Early positive end-expiratory pressure in adult respiratory distress syndrome. Arch Surg 114:497–501

Williamson DC III, Modell JH (1982) Intermittent continuous positive airway pressure by mask. Arch Surg 118:970–972

Zebrowsky ME, Geer RT (1981) Low field continuous positive airway pressure with a modified fresh gas reservoir. Crit Care Med 9:106–108

Pressure Support Ventilation

L. Brochard and G. Iotti

In recent years various modalities of partial ventilatory support have evolved in the care of critically ill patients, which are tending to replace fully controlled mechanical ventilation (CMV). At least three reasons explain this development.

In patients under mechanical ventilation, spontaneous inspiratory activity is still present except in the case of respiratory muscle fatigue or excessive loading for the respiratory muscles (Rochester et al. 1977), hypocapnic hyperventilation, central nervous system disorders, or administration of sedative drugs. Therefore, new modes of mechanical ventilation have been developed which allow spontaneous breathing by the patient with optimal ventilator synchrony. These modes of ventilation also reduce the need for sedation.

Prolonged periods of complete respiratory muscle rest may lead to atrophy due to disuse. Maintenance of some spontaneous activity is thus probably preferable in preparation for the weaning phase.

During weaning from mechanical ventilation, the use of such modes has become widespread for patients experiencing difficulty in tolerating discontinuation of mechanical ventilation.

Pressure support ventilation (PSV) seems to be a very promising alternative for use during the weaning phase. This is because during assist-control ventilation or synchronized intermittent mandatory ventilation (SIMV) excessive respiratory muscle work may be performed by the patients. Indeed this is one of the main criticisms of these modes. During the assist-control mode, the patient does not cease respiratory effort with the onset of the triggered breath. Significant exertion of the respiratory musculature persists throughout each patient-initiated ventilator cycle, often at levels taxing the ventilatory reserve (Marini et al. 1986). SIMV allows the patient to continue to breathe spontaneously with only intermittent supplementation from the ventilator. However, spontaneous breaths occur through demand valve systems which may impose additional work and excessive work of breathing has been documented during this mode of ventilation (Weisman et al. 1983). While these modalities of ventilation are reliable under most circumstances, excessive work can preclude successful weaning in patients in whom the respiratory muscles are stressed near to the point of fatigue (Cohen et al. 1982). PSV, which was designed to decrease the work of breathing, may be of special interest in these cases.

Operational Principles

During PSV, a constant positive pressure is applied to the airways during the inspiratory phase of each patient's triggered breath (Fig. 1). There is no preset tidal volume and cycles are flow limited and not pressure limited. The patient controls the respiratory rate, inspiratory and expiratory time, and tidal volume, while the ventilator supplies assistance to each breath. However, the setting of the ventilator may interfere with the pattern of breathing of the patient. The degree of assistance is regulated by the level of pressure support delivered with each breath.

For regular use, the variables which must be set are:

1. The trigger level (in cm H_2O below positive end expiratory pressure, PEEP). The trigger must therefore be set at a low level to reduce the inspiratory effort of the patient (maximal sensitivity).
2. The pressure support (PS) level (0–30 or 60 cm H_2O, depending on the ventilator).
3. Because on the principles upon which PSV works neither volume nor frequency settings can be used.

Respiratory Cycle Periods

The method by which intermittent pressure support (IPS) operates varies markedly according to the different sytems available. Three events can be distinguished during a complete breath under PSV.

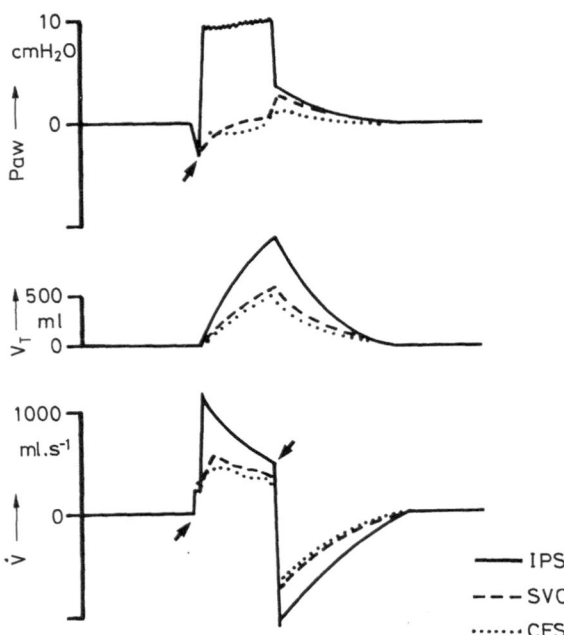

Fig. 1. Diagram of airway pressure (Paw), tidal volume (V_t), and flow ($\dot{V}$) during three modes of ventilatory assistance: inspiratory pressure support (IPS), spontaneous breathing through the Siemens Servo 900 C circuit (SVC) or through a continuous flow system (CFS). Opening of the demand valve is indicated with an *arrow* on the pressure trace. With IPS a plateau of pressure is produced during the entire inspiration (*arrows* on flow delineate pressure support time). (From Brochard et al. 1987)

Triggering of Inspiration. This is initiated by the inspiratory effort of the patient and is usually detected by a pressure sensor. The trigger sensitivity is either fixed or (usually) adjustable. This mechanism requires an effort which in the past has been reported to impede the patient's inspiratory effort, but now modern demand valves are of better quality and have shorter time responses. One ventilator (Engströem Erica) triggers inspiration on flow demand instead of pressure. The opening time delay varies between 50 and 150 ms depending upon the ventilator and published data are available in the literature (Cox et al. 1988). Though studies specifically concerning PSV are lacking, there is general agreement that, whenever respiratory cycles are patient-initiated, a high sensitivity of the trigger, together with a fast time response of the ventilator allows a reduction of the work of breathing (Kacmarek 1988) and better comfort for the patient. Obviously, sensitivity must not be so high as to cause self-cycling.

Inspiration. Once inspiration has been initiated the ventilator delivers a high inspiratory flow which decreases throughout the whole period of inspiration. The servoregulatory mechanism maintains the proper flow necessary to reach the appropriate preset pressure support level and maintains it constant until expiration occurs. The flow regulation varies between the different ventilators and it determines the exact pressure wave form. In a relaxed patient, a square wave is obtained by an exponential decreasing flow. Instantaneous pressure and flow thus depend upon the time constant of the respiratory system (determined by compliance and resistance) and on the initial flow generated by the ventilator. If the pressure is maintained at a plateau, the tidal volume will result from the product of the total compliance and the inflation pressure (IPS level minus total PEEP).

Pressurization Rate. Pressure increases according to a rate that is system-specific and generally nonadjustable. A high pressurization rate results in a square pressure wave, while a low pressurization rate results in a more progressive achievement of the preset pressure support level. Only few ventilators (Siemens Servoventilator 900 C, Dräger EV–A and EVITA) allow setting of this parameter.

The pressurization rate has been shown to influence the ventilatory pattern (Braschi et al. 1989). A low pressurization rate is disadvantageous since it may excessively increase the inspiration time/total time ratio (T_i/T_{tot}). This is true at least for ventilators whose expiratory trigger sensitivity is dependent on the inspiratory peak flow (see below). On the other hand, a high pressurization rate induces a value of T_i/T_{tot} lower than 0.5. The resulting square wave should be also more efficacious from the standpoint of assistance to the patient, although it can be associated with a reduction of tidal volume in extreme situations. We recently showed that the "fast" pressure wave had a greater efficacy than the "slow" one to reduce the work of breathing (Messadi et al. 1990).

For any inspiratory effort the addition of pressure support augments the pressure difference between the circuit and the alveoli, leading to a higher inspiratory flow rate and a higher tidal volume than during spontaneous breathing.

Thus, whatever the IPS level may be this mode always increases the inspiratory flow rate of the patient in a way which remains under patient regulation. This characteristic differs strikingly from all the other ventilatory modes. During the assist-control mode, the inspiratory effort of the patient leads only to a reduction in the ventilator work but does not modify either flow or volume; if the required flow becomes greater than the flow supplied by the ventilator, the patient will exhaust his inspiratory effort without any resulting increase in tidal volume.

Triggering of Expiration. Three criteria allow recognition of the expiration phase. During PSV the cycling to exhalation is triggered by a decrease of the inspiratory flow from the peak to a system-specific threshold value. This critical decrease of the inspiratory flow is a signal that the inspiratory muscles have begun to relax. The threshold value for cycling, that represents the sensitivity of the expiratory trigger, is nonadjustable. According to the ventilator, it is either an absolute level of flow (between 2 and 6 l/min) or a fixed percentage of the peak (25% or 12%).

Braschi et al. (1989) investigated the effects of different expiratory trigger sensitivities using a modified ventilator provided with a high pressurization rate and a selection of different percentages of sensitivity. From their study, it was concluded that the optimal sensitivity for a ventilator is a function of the pressurization rate. A combination of high pressurization rate and low sensitivity of the expiratory trigger appears to be the most advantageous setting. On the other hand, if a low pressurization rate has been chosen, a high sensitivity seems to be the only way to prevent an excessive increase of T_i/T_{tot}. Moreover, different categories of patients could benefit from different values of sensitivity. For instance, if we consider the effect on T_i/T_{tot}, a low sensitivity could be indicated for restrictive patients, while a high one could be more adapted for obstructive patients. Therefore, there could be some interest in having the opportunity to adjust the expiratory sensitivity.

The detection of a small degree of pressure (1–3 cm H_2O) above the fixed IPS level is the second criterion allowing recognition of the expiratory phase. In theory this should necessitate a sudden expiratory effort by the patient and could lengthen the inspiratory time. However, this may not necessarily be detrimental, since an end inspiratory plateau has been reported to increase the oxygenation. On the other hand, it may require repeated extra expiratory muscular work. This criterion is frequently associated with the first one.

Finally, as part of the control of PSV, a time limit for inspiration is usually added. This works as a safety mechanism so that whenever a leak is present in the circuit the two previous systems become inoperative. Hazards have been reported in the absence of this device when constant insufflation at the PSV level has created high continuous positive airway pressure (CPAP) levels (Black and Grover 1988).

Changes in Breathing Pattern During PSV

Several investigators have focused on the changes in breathing pattern during PSV (MacIntyre 1986; Ershowsky and Krieger 1987; Brochard et al. 1987, 1989). When compared with unaided spontaneous breathing, the addition of pressure support increases the tidal volume and decreases respiratory rate. With increasing levels of pressure support a gradual increase in volume and reduction in rate are observed. This reduced respiratory rate can help to reduce any intrinsic PEEP resulting from reduction of the expiratory time and thus reducing lung hyperinflation. Minute ventilation is generally stable due to the combined effects of an increase in tidal volume and a reduction of the breathing frequency. However, in hypercapnic acidotic patients, the minute ventilation may increase initially when changing from the purely spontaneous mode of breathing to assisted ventilation with PS and then remain stable for higher levels of pressure support.

In patients with deteriorating gaseous exchange during spontaneous breathing, i.e., hypoxemia and hypercapnia, the arterial blood gas tensions may be improved by the addition of pressure support, thus allowing the patient to regulate his respiratory activity at a lower $PaCO_2$.

Respiratory Muscle Work

A recent study investigated the effects of PSV on the mechanical work of breathing, oxygen cost of breathing, and diaphragmatic activity (Brochard et al. 1989). In eight patients with difficulty in tolerating discontinuation from mechanical ventilation despite adequate therapy, several levels of PSV were compared, from 0 (i.e., spontaneous breathing without assistance) to 20 cm H_2O of pressure support. During PS 0 the patients exhibited a characteristic pattern of breathing, with small tidal volumes at a high rate. This has been found to be associated with unsuccessful weaning (Tobin et al. 1986). This particular pattern was accompanied by a decrease in PaO_2 and a significant increase in $PaCO_2$. In the same period, patients performed high levels of work of breathing and the oxygen cost of breathing was estimated to be as high as 25% of the total oxygen consumption. Diaphragmatic electromyogram (EMG) studies were recorded and the ratio of high frequency components to low frequency components of the diaphragmatic electromyogram (H/L) was measured as an index of impending diaphragmatic fatigue. During PS 0 seven of the eight patients exhibited marked signs of diaphragmatic fatigue, a finding which explained their inability to be weaned from the ventilator. Pressure support was then delivered at 10, 15, and 20 cm H_2O. Concomitant with increasing levels of PSV, alterations in breathing pattern and arterial blood gases were observed, as described above. A dramatic reduction in the work of breathing performed by the patients, the oxygen cost of breathing, and diaphragmatic activity were also demonstrated (Fig. 2). The magnitude of the work was inversely correlated with the level of pressure support

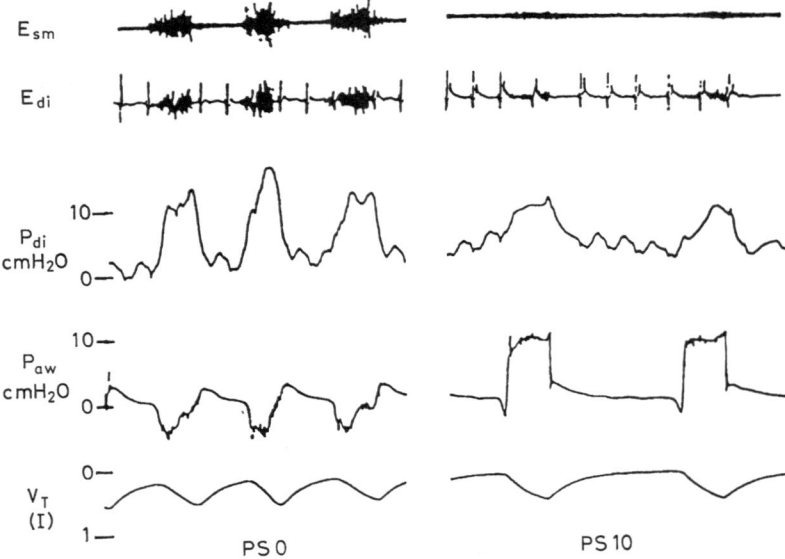

E_{sm}

E_{di}

P_{di}
cmH_2O
10—
0—

P_{aw}
cmH_2O
10—
0—

V_T
(I)
0—
1—

PS 0   PS 10

Fig. 2. Recordings of electrical activity of the sternocleidomastoid muscle (Esm) and of the diaphragm (Edi), transdiaphragmatic pressure (Pdi), airway pressure (Paw), and tidal volume (V t) for a patient without inspiratory pressure support (*PS 0*) and with 10 cm H_2O of pressure support (*PS 10*). Note the dramatic decrease in respiratory muscle activity, the increased tidal volume, and the decreased respiratory rate during PS 10. (From Brochard et al. 1989)

delivered. Diaphragmatic activity, although always present, was progressively reduced. In addition the EMG signs of diaphragmatic fatigue were suppressed at 10 cm H_2O in four patients and at 20 cm H_2O in three patients. In another study performed in postoperative patients without preexisting pulmonary disease, 15 cm H_2O PSV was shown to take over the major part of the work of breathing assessed by the oxygen cost of breathing (Viale et al. 1988). Thus, by setting the pressure level adequately, the physician may regulate the work of breathing of the patient and find an optimal work load for the respiratory muscles.

Pressure Support Level

The tidal volume is, in part, dependent upon the mechanical characteristics of the respiratory system. As a result PSV may have two effects. First, high levels of pressure support may result in very large tidal volume being delivered which may be followed by periods of apnea. Second, for an identical level of pressure support any modification of the mechanical characteristics of the respiratory system will change the resulting tidal volume for an identical inspiratory effort, or it may impose additional work for the patient to maintain the same tidal volume. This may lead to the need to modify the setting of the ventilator at this time.

One of the problems associated with this mode of ventilatory support is to find the "optimum level" of pressure support for each patient. A suboptimal level may be insufficient to assist the respiratory muscles during a fatiguing pattern, while an excessively high level may be responsible for potentially dangerous hyperinflation. A simple method is to set up the appropriate PSV level, giving enough pressure support to obtain a predetermined tidal volume (for instance, 10 ml/kg tidal volume). Another method is to set an arbitrary optimal breathing frequency, which can vary from 10 to 25 breaths per minute, depending upon the clinician.

The optimum level of pressure support can also be defined ideally as the lowest level required to maintain diaphragmatic activity without fatigue (Brochard et al. 1989). A simple means of assessing this level is to monitor sternocleidomastoid muscle activity. The electrical muscular activity of this particular muscle, one of the auxiliary muscles of inspiration, is greater when the diaphragm is fatigued. The activation of the sternomastoid muscle is to due to an increased demand for ventilation. PSV decreases the activity of the sternomastoid by decreasing the work of breathing. At the optimum pressure support level, the sternomastoid has minimal activity. Thus, monitoring of PSV could be done at the bedside by palpating the muscular activity of the sternomastoid. Pressure support should be diminished progressively from high levels such as 30 cm H_2O until the phasic inspiratory activity of the sterno-mastoid appears to increase; at this point 5 cm H_2O more pressure support should be added.

Servocontroling the pressure support level is an interesting way to resolve the question of the adequate level of pressure and its modification over time. This is offered by several ventilators and the controlled value is either minute ventilation or the breathing frequency of the patient. This last modality seems to be an interesting and promising mode of partial ventilatory support (Boyer et al. 1989).

Suppression of the Extra Work Induced by the Endotracheal Tube

Several authors have proposed that PSV could be used to suppress the extra work of breathing induced by the presence of an endotracheal tube (Fiastro et al. 1988; Brochard et al. 1988). In addition, the presence of a demand valve and the ventilator circuitry induces a supplemental load which can be overcome by a certain amount of PSV. The work of breathing spontaneously before and after extubation has been measured (Brochard et al. 1988). Breathing through the endotracheal tube was found to induce a significant extra workload. This extra work was much higher in a group of six patients with chronic lung disease (nearly 40% of the work obtained after extubation) compared with five patients free of lung disease in whom the extra work was virtually negligible (13% of the work measured after extubation). The pressure support level necessary to suppress this extra work was always above 8 cm H_2O. Thus, in patients with chronic lung disease, who represent most of the difficult-to-wean patients, tolerance of a pressure support level less than 8 cm H_2O for at least 24 h probably indicates that extubation can be performed without risks of excessive respiratory muscle work. In patients free of lung disease, however, much lower levels of pressure support are able to suppress the extra work induced by the tube.

Differences with Intermittent Positive Pressure Breathing (IPPB)

Some similarities exist between IPPB and PSV. In both methods the ventilatory cycles are triggered by the patient and neither deliver volume controlled ventilation. However, during PSV the flow is usually decelerating, while in IPPB the flow is either constant or decelerating. In IPPB circuits the pressure delivered depends upon both the flow supplied and the patient's demand as there is no servocontrolled loop present to regulate pressure. Thus, with IPPB in case of active inspiration the pressure in the circuit can become negative thereby imposing an external workload on the patient because of the imbalance between supply and demand. In contrast, during PSV the inspiratory pressure is maintained constant, at least theoretically, by adjustment of the flow according to the patient's demand, thus allowing a decrease in the work of breathing.

Further differences exist in that with IPPB the cycles are pressure limited whereas they are mainly flow limited with PSV. This pressure limitation with IPPB can lead to an active expiratory effort being required in order to reach the pressure level which triggers expiration. This is different from PSV. The work of breathing in healthy volunteers has been measured recently during CO_2-induced hyperventilation with both PSV and IPPB (Mancebo et al. 1988). In such conditions of high ventilatory demand induced by CO_2-induced hyperventilation, the differences in workload between the two methods were considerable. A large extra workload was measured with IPPB compared with PSV. Only PSV was able to decrease the work of breathing during these conditions of high ventilatory demand.

Clinical Applications

IPS increases markedly the efficacy of spontaneous breathing under these circumstances while reducing the activity of the inspiratory muscles. The ventilator-patient synchrony is good since the respiratory rate is determined by the patient, and, as each breath is efficiently assisted, this enables the patient to breathe spontaneously for sustained periods. Sophisticated monitoring of ventilation is performed by ventilators offering the pressure support mode. However, there is no evidence to date that PSV can shorten the weaning time or reduce complications related to mechanical ventilation. Thus, indications for pressure support can not yet be defined clearly and are still a matter of individual choice.

However, several factors favour the use of PSV in certain circumstances. The hemodynamic status seems to be similar during PSV and other modes of ventilatory support (Fargier et al. 1987; Prakash and Meij 1985). Several authors have reported that patients felt more comfortable during PSV than during CPAP or assisted mechanical ventilation (AMV), although this evidence is based on subjective criteria. Another study in postoperative patients has shown that the arterial blood gases were improved in PSV compared with AMV despite a lower minute ventilation; in addition, these patients required less sedation (Fargier et al. 1987). Patients experiencing difficulties in weaning from mechanical ventilation may well benefit from the use of pressure support ventilation which can also be used as a ventilatory support mode without the need for sedation. However, when sedation is needed, or if the respiratory muscles require complete rest, or if a decrease in oxygen consumption is sought, then PSV appears to be contraindicated. Similarly, PSV should not be used in patients with central neurological disorders and no ventilatory drive.

Conclusion

Inspiratory pressure support (IPS) has been shown, in short-term studies, to offer several major advantages and to be beneficial for patients. One advantage (not reported) is that IPS can also be delivered via a face mask in nonintubated patients. Such "physiological assistance" may be indicated for patients where intermittent positive pressure breathing would be inappropriate and in other cases as a means to avoid intubation (Brochard et al. 1990). Long-term studies during weaning from mechanical ventilation are clearly needed to precisely define the still putative advantages of this method.

References

Black JW, Grover BS (1988) A hazard of pressure support ventilation. Chest 93:333–335
Boyer F, Bruneau B, Gaussorgues P, Jay-Lassonnery S, Robert D (1989) Aide inspiratoire avec asservissement du niveau de pression: volume ventilé minute versus fréquence ventilatoire. Reanim Soins Intensive Med Urgence 5:227–232
Braschi A, Rodi G, Sala Gallini G, Iotti G, Chiaranda M (1989) Relationships between pressurization rate and breathing pattern during pressure support ventilation (Abstr). Am Rev Respir Dis 139:A155
Braschi A, Sala Gallini G, Rodi G, Iotti G, Chiaranda M, Villa S (1989) Relationships between sensitivity of the expiratory trigger and breathing pattern during pressure support ventilation (Abstr). Am Rev Respir Dis 139:A361
Brochard L, Pluskwa F, Lemaire F (1987) Improved efficacy of spontaneous breathing with inspiratory pressure support. Am Rev Respir Dis 32:1011–1016
Brochard L, Rua F, Lorino H, Lemaire F, Harf A (1988) Suppression of the extra work of breathing due to the endotracheal tube with inspiratory pressure support. Am Rev Respir Dis 137:A64

Brochard L, Harf A, Lorino H, Lemaire F (1989) Inspiratory pressure support prevents diaphragmatic fatigue during weaning from mechanical ventilation. Am Rev Respir Dis 139:513–521
Brochard L, Isabey D, Piquet J, Amaro P, Mancebo J, Messadi AA, Brun-Buisson C, Rauss A, Lemaire F, Harf A (1990) Reversal of acute exacerbations of chronic obstructive lung disease by inspiratory assistance with a face mask. N Engl J Med 323:1523–30
Cohen CA, Zagelbaum G, Gross D, Roussos C, Macklem PT (1982) Clinical manifestations of inspiratory muscle fatigue. Am J Med 73:308–316
Cox D, Tinloi SF, Farrimond JG (1988) Investigation of the spontaneous modes of breathing of different ventilators. Intensive Care Med 14:532–537
Ershowsky P, Krieger B (1987) Changes in breathing pattern during pressure support ventilation. Respir Care 32:1011–1016
Fargier JJ, Robert D, Boyer F, Chagny J, Kopp C, Baulieux J, Moskovtchenko JF, Pouyet M (1987) Positive pressure inspiratory aid vs assisted mechanical ventilation after esophageal Surgery. J Crit Care 2:101–108
Fiastro JF, Habib MP, Quan SF (1988) Pressure support compensation for inspiratory work due to endotracheal tubes and demand continuous positive airway pressure. Chest 93:499–505
Kacmarek RM (1988) The role of pressure support ventilation in reducing work of breathing. Respir Care 33:99–120
MacIntyre NR (1986) Respiratory function during pressure support ventilation. Chest 89:677–683
Mancebo J, Brochard L, Amaro R, Mollo JL, Harf A, Lemaire F (1988) Is inspiratory pressure support similar to intermittent positive breathing? Intensive Care Med 14:A326
Marini JJ, Rodriguez RM, Lamb V (1986) The inspiratory workload of patient-initiated mechanical ventilation. Am Rev Respir Dis 132:902–909
Messadi AA, Ben Ayed M, Brochard L, Iotti G, Harf A, Lemaire F (1990) Comparison of the efficacy of two waveforms of inspiratory pressure support: slow versus fast pressure wave. Am Rev Respir Dis 141:A519
Prakash O, Meij S (1985) Cardiopulmonary response to inspiratory pressure support during spontaneous ventilation vs conventional ventilation. Chest 88:403–408
Rochester DF, Braun NMT, Laine S (1977) Diaphragmatic energy expenditure in chronic respiratory failure. The effect of assisted ventilation with body respirator. Am J Med 63:223–231
Tobin MJ, Perez W, Guenther SH, Semmes BJ, Mador MJ, Allen SJ, Lodato RF, Dantzker DR (1986) The pattern of breathing during successful and unsuccessful trials of weaning from mechanical ventilation. Am Rev Respir Dis 134:1111–1118
Viale JP, Annat GJ, Bouffard YM, Delafosse BX, Bertrand OH, Motin JP (1988) Oxygen cost of breathing in post-operative patients. Chest 93:506–509
Weisman IM, Rinaldo JE, Rogers RM, Sanders MH (1983) Intermittent mandatory ventilation. Am Rev Respir Dis 127:641–647

Mandatory Minute Volume Ventilation

J.-P. Laaban, M. Ben Ayed, and M.-J. Fevrier

Principle of Operation

Mandatory minute volume ventilation (MMV) is an original mode of mechanical ventilation introduced by Hewlett et al. in 1977. In this mode, the patient is guaranteed a predetermined (expired) minute volume (V_E), called the preset minute volume. If the patient is able to spontaneously breathe sufficiently to fit the preset minute volume, the ventilator does not deliver any mechanical breath. If the patient is unable to breathe spontaneously, the ventilator delivers mechanical breaths so that the patient receives a minute volume equal to the preset V_E. If the spontaneous breathing of the patient is inferior to the preset V_E, the remainder is automatically provided by the ventilator. The values of the preset V_E and of the mechanical tidal volume (V_T) are predetermined. The adjustments of the mechanical ventilation according to the changes in spontaneous breathing are usually (CPU 1) achieved by a modification of the rate of mechanical breaths. If the spontaneous ventilation exceeds the preset V_E, the ventilator progressively decreases the frequency of mechanical breaths and can possibly stop delivering mechanical ventilation. Conversely, if the spontaneous ventilation is less than the preset V_E, the ventilator progressively increases the rate of mechanical breaths. If no spontaneous breathing is present, all of the preset V_E will be provided by the ventilator with a frequency of mechanical breaths equal to the ratio of the preset V_E to V_T. With this mode of ventilatory support, the rate of mandatory breaths automatically changes according to the variations in the ability of the patient to breathe (Fig. 1). This ventilatory mode which combines spontaneous breaths and mechanical breaths is close to the intermittent mandatory ventilation (IMV). With IMV, the ventilator tidal volume and respiratory rate are predetermined and spontaneous breaths are permitted between mechanical breaths. However, if IMV is used with a low rate of mandatory breaths, any depression of spontaneous breathing (for instance, following injection of sedative drugs) may result in an alveolar hypoventilation with severe respiratory acidosis. Alveolar hypoventilation should not occur with MMV, at least if the preset V_E is high enough, because the patient is ensured to receive the preset V_E even if his spontaneous ventilation is markedly depressed. The selection of the preset V_E is of great importance: a low preset V_E will be associated with a mainly spontaneous ventilatory mode, but alveolar hypoventilation may occur. Conversely, with too high a preset V_E that largely

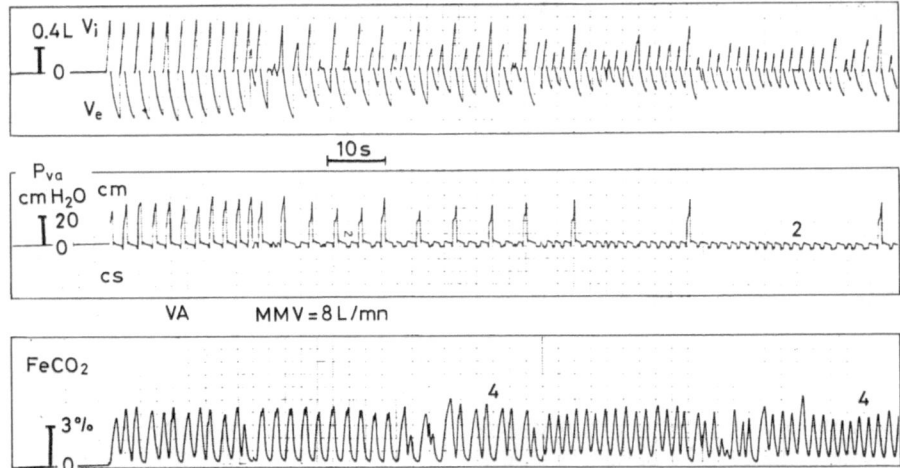

Fig. 1. Variation of the ventilatory mode in MMV. The rate of mechanical cycles progressively decreases so that the patient's ventilatory mode is mostly spontaneous. Indeed, the patient's spontaneous ventilation exceeds the preset minute volume ($V_E = 8$ l/min). V_i, inspired tidal volume; V_e, expired tidal volume; P_{va}, airways pressure; CM, mechanical cycle; CS, spontaneous cycle; $FeCO_2$, end-expiratory CO_2 concentration

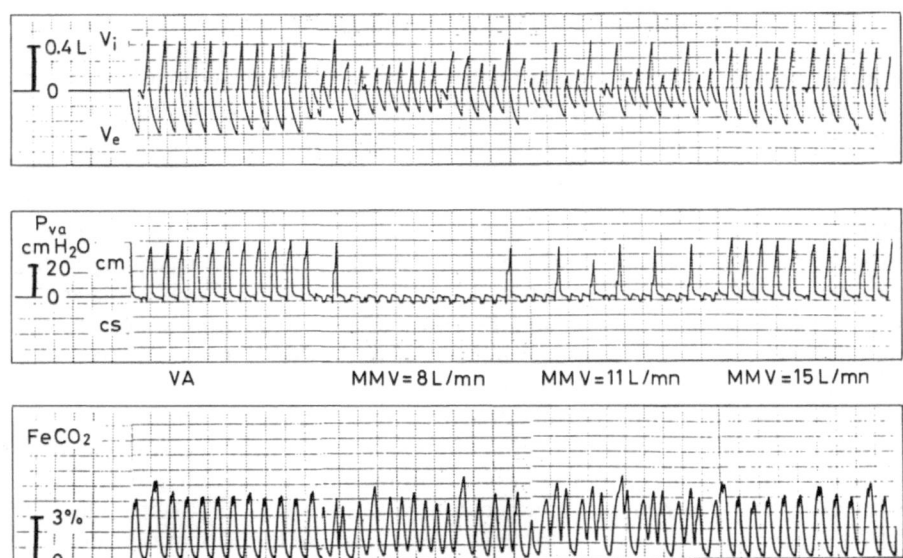

Fig. 2. Influence of the MMV volume on the respiratory mode in patients under MMV. If the V_E is equal to 8 l/min, the ventilatory mode is mostly spontaneous. If V_E has a much higher value (15 l/min), the ventilation is solely mechanical. Mechanical and spontaneous cycles are associated with an intermediate V_E (11 l/min). Va, assisted ventilation

exceeds the patient's ability to breathe spontaneously, the ventilatory mode will be purely mechanical. Variations of the ventilatory mode in a given patient under MMV with different preset V_E are shown in Fig. 2.

Ventilators Providing MMV

Several ventilators, available at present, can provide MMV, including the CPU 1 (Ohmeda), Erica (Engström), EVA (Dräger), Bear-5, and Veolar (Hamilton).

CPU 1. The V_E (including spontaneous and mechanical breaths) in the CPU 1 is compared every 24 cycles with the preset V_E. The period between two mechanical breaths is progressively and automatically adjusted in order to reduce the difference between expired V_E and preset V_E. The ventilator modifies the frequency of mechanical breaths by changing the expiration time. The progressive decrease of mechanical cycles from a completely mechanical ventilatory mode to nearly completely spontaneous breathing takes about 16 min (Nunn and Lyle 1986). The same algorithm is available in the ADVENT.

Positive end expiratory pressure (PEEP) can be associated to the MMV mode, as well as inspiratory pressure support.

Erica The Erica microprocessor measures the V_E for the last 30 s, compares it with the preset V_E on a breath-by-breath basis, and determines the duration of the zero-flow periods (apnea). The principle of MMV with the Erica is to allow complete spontaneous breathing aided as required by one or more mechanical cycles. If the expired V_E is inferior to the present V_E, the ventilator delivers a tidal volume (V_T) equal to the preset V_T and this may be repeated as long as V_E remains below the preset value.

Provided the expired V_E exceeds the preset V_E, the following modes of support will apply: (a) when the patient's spontaneous breathing is regular, no mechanical cycle is provided; (b) when the patient's spontaneous breathing is irregular (i.e., with periods of apnea), a "time limitation" function will prevent the occurrence of protracted apnea. Thus, when the patient's spontaneous breathing is suppressed during a period exceeding $60 \times (V_T + 0.2)/V_E$ s, the ventilator will provide a mechanical breath. The modifications of the mechanical ventilation according to the patient's ability to breathe spontaneously are faster than with CPU 1. PEEP and pressure support may be added to the spontaneous breaths.

Veolar The MMV differs from the other MMV systems because modifications of the level of pressure support ensure that the patient receives a minute volume at least equal to the preset V_E. The ventilator calculates the V_E averaged on the eight last breaths and compares V_E with the preset V_E on a breath-by-breath basis. If V_E is inferior to the preset V_E, the ventilator increases the level of pressure support by 2 or 3 cm H_2O. On the other hand, if V_E exceeds the preset V_E, the level of pressure support is automatically decreased by 2 or 3 cm H_2O. The value of pressure support ranges from 2 to 30 cm H_2O above the PEEP level. A safety setting allows the IMV mode to resume automatically in the event of an apnea

MMV VEOLAR

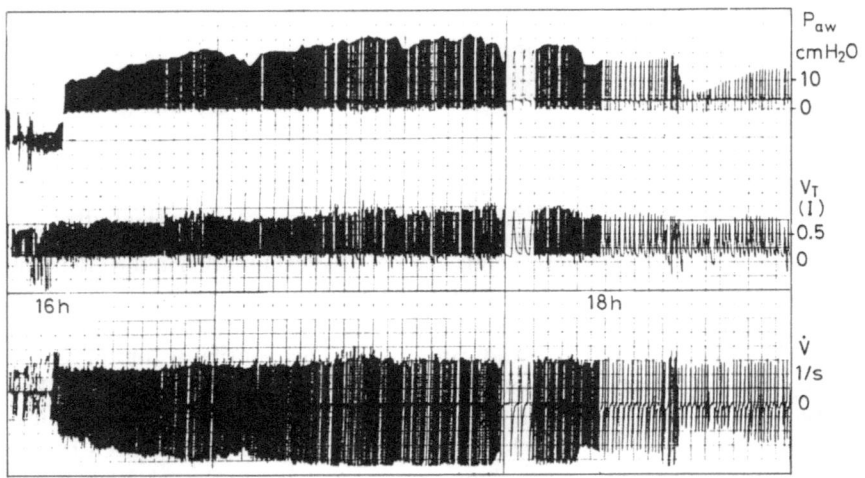

Preset vent.8 L/mn

Fig. 3. Veolar MMV. Airway pressure (PAw), tidal volume (V_T), and flow ($\dot{V}$) tracings in a 45-year-old female patient undergoing MMV ventilation (Veolar) with a preset V_E equal to 8 l/min. One can notice the variations of the pressure support from 0 cm H_2O (*right part of the tracing*) to 20 cm H_2O (*middle part of the tracing*, around 5 pm). (From Lemaire et al. 1983)

which is equal or superior to 5 s. Ben Ayed et al. (1986) have shown in ten patients that the Veolar MMV may be an interesting method for weaning patients from ventilatory support, especially those with small tidal volumes during spontaneous breathing (Fig. 3).

A New Approach: Pressure Support Mandatory Minute Frequency Recently, Boyer et al. (1988a) proposed a new way of performing MMV: a preset respiratory rate range is selected, and then the ventilator adjusts the level of inspiratory pressure support (IPS) to fit that target, using the principle that high levels of IPS to fit that target, using the principle that high levels of IPS reduce the spontaneous respiratory rate. By increasing the dead space by 300 ml in seven spontaneously breathing intensive care patients, Boyer et al. (1988b) showed their new form of MMV enabled the patients to increase V_E without producing hyperpnea; the increased level of pressure support augmented each tidal breath. This mode is provided by the CESAR (Air Liquide).

Monitoring of MMV

The main characteristic of MMV is its great flexibility in allowing the ventilatory mode of the patient to change from being fully spontaneous to being partly spontaneous-partly mechanical or to complete mechanical ventilation. The monitoring system must allow a separate analysis of spontaneous and mechanical breaths. However, only very close supervision can help to determine which ventilatory mode is predominant over a 24-h period. The ideal monitoring system should be able to record ventilation continuously while the data are stocked into a microcomputer. A report on the ventilatory parameters over the past 24 h could thereby be provided detailing modes of total ventilation, spontaneous ventilation, and mechanical ventilation. Thus, the respective percentages of spontaneous and mechanical breathing over 24 h could be determined (Ohmeda monitor).

Advantages of MMV

It has been suggested that MMV, like IMV, by maintaining spontaneous breathing, prevents the atrophy of respiratory muscles that develops after prolonged mechanical ventilatory assistance (Weisman et al. 1983). The atrophy of respiratory muscles may be enhanced by malnutrition or sepsis, resulting in a decrease of the strength of inspiratory muscles that would prolong the weaning from mechanical ventilation. In patients under prolonged mechanical ventilation respiratory muscle discoordination and asynchrony have been described, resulting in ineffective spontaneous breathing and lengthening of the weaning phase. Thus, maintaining spontaneous breathing could represent respiratory muscle "training" which might prevent atrophy and discoordination of respiratory muscles. Theoretically, this objective can be achieved with both IMV and MMV. However, it has not been shown that IMV is superior to periods of spontaneous T-piece breathing in this regard (Cameron and Oh 1986). Indeed, short periods of spontaneous T-piece breathing with added inspiratory resistive loads may be more efficient than MMV in increasing the strength and endurance of respiratory muscles (Sonne and Davis 1982).

The major advantage of MMV over IMV is *safety*. Irrespective of the ability of the patient to breathe spontaneously, the delivery of the preset V_E will always be guaranteed with MMV. With IMV, however, alveolar hypoventilation may develop if the patient's spontaneous ventilation decreases, for example, if there is a decline in the neurological status. Moreover, if the patient is unable to increase his spontaneous respiration to meet an increase in ventilatory requirements, hypercapnia may ensue using the IMV mode if the rate of mechanical breaths is too low. Covelli et al. (1981) reported three observations of patients with chronic lung disease receiving ventilatory support with IMV who developed severe hypercapnia several hours after the onset of a hypercaloric parenteral nutrition; indeed, these patients were unable to increase their spontaneous ventilation adequately to meet the rise in CO_2 production induced by the high carbohydrate load.

The use of MMV is said to reduce the supervision required during the weaning process. Indeed, during periods of spontaneous T-piece breathing, the presence of a nurse or a physiotherapist is absolutely necessary to detect signs of alveolar hypoventilation and reconnect the patient to the ventilator. On the other hand, in the MMV mode, if the patient becomes rapidly exhausted with a marked decrease of spontaneous ventilation, the preset V_E is automatically delivered by the ventilator.

The use of MMV may be associated with several advantages that have been claimed but not clearly demonstrated for IMV:

1. Diminished likelihood of respiratory alkalosis (Benzer 1982) (however, a respiratory alkalosis may develop with the MMV mode if the preset V_E exceeds the patient's ventilatory demands.
2. Less need for sedatives and muscle relaxants to achieve ventilator synchrony.
3. More uniform intrapulmonary gas distribution.
4. Lower mean airway pressure with a reduced risk of barotrauma (Mathru et al. 1983) and less cardiovascular depression.

Disadvantages of MMV

The major risk associated with the MMV mode is the development of severe hypercapnia in patients with a spontaneous breathing pattern characterized by a high respiratory rate and a low tidal volume that is virtually equal to the dead

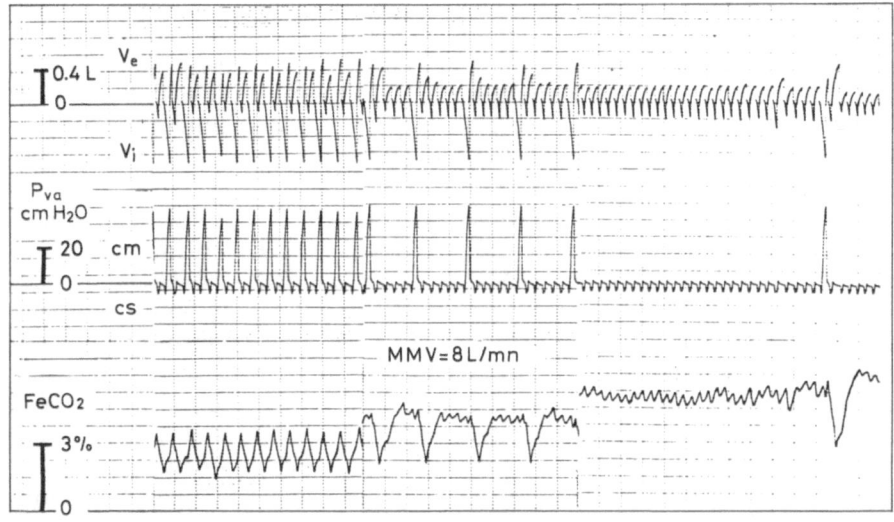

Fig. 4. Risk of alveolar hypoventilation due to rapid shallow breathing in MMV. Tracing of a 60-year-old female patient with an extensive bacterial pneumonia. The patient's spontaneous ventilation (9.4 l/min) exceeds the preset V_E (8 l/min), so that the ventilator stops delivering mechanical breaths. But this spontaneous breathing is ineffective with a tidal volume of 180 ml and a respiratory rate of 52 breaths/min. Arterial blood gas analysis reveals a severe respiratory acidosis ($PaCO_2$, 84 mmHg; PaO_2, 45 mmHg; pH, 7.10)

space (shallow breathing). Indeed, if the patient's spontaneous ventilation with these rapid shallow breaths exceeds the preset V_E, the ventilator stops delivering mechanical breaths in spite of the fact that the spontaneous breathing is ineffective. This may result in severe alveolar hypoventilatin with marked hypercapnia (Fig. 4). Thus, a safety setting is mandatory in ventilators providing MMV, so that mechanical ventilation is automatically resumed if the spontaneous ventilation is ineffective with rapid shallow breaths. Several systems have been proposed, including the following:

1. Alarm for minimal tidal volume. This safety setting is present in the CPU1. If the tidal volume (averaged on five breaths) is inferior to a preselected value, the ventilator automatically delivers a mechanical ventilation equal to the preset V_E; 1/4 or 3/8 of the mechanical tidal volume (V_T) may be selected as inadequate. Selecting 3/8 V_T offers a greater safety than 1/4 V_T, but patients with relatively small tidal volumes will experience some difficulty to maintain a spontaneous ventilatory mode (Fig. 5).

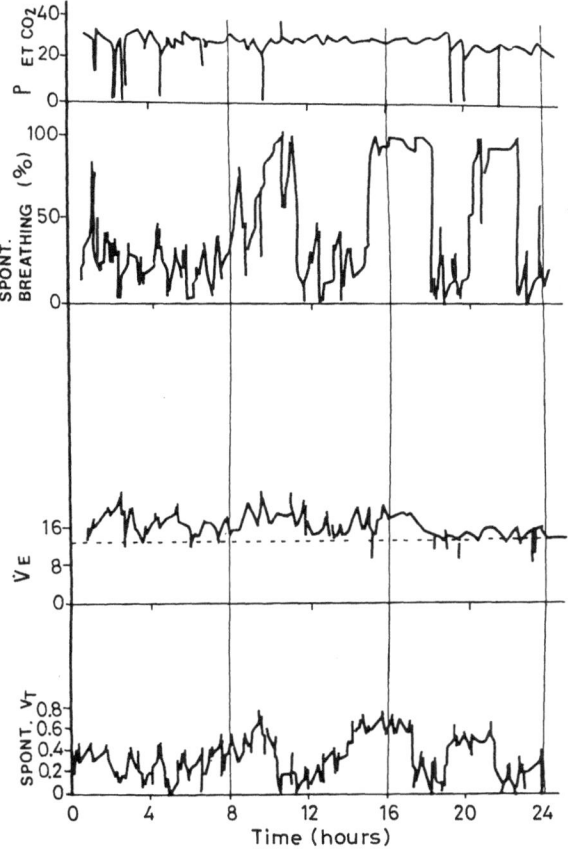

Fig. 5. A 24-h recording during MMV ventilation (CPU1) in a patient with Guillain-Barré syndrome. During the 24 h displayed, $P_{ET}CO_2$ remained stable at about 30 mmHg, indicating efficient ventilation was achieved with both spontaneous and mechanical ventilation. V_E remained at the MMV level during mechanical ventilation but was higher during spontaneous ventilation. *Lower trace* shows that the spontaneous tidal volume (spont V_T) slowly increased to 0.5 l, allowing unaided spontaneous ventilation. Then, as the patient fatigued, spontaneous ventilation decreased sharply while mechanical breathing resumed. $P_{ET}CO_2$, end tidal CO_2 (mmHg)

2. Rate alarm for tachypnea. This alarm is provided in the Erica so that mechanical ventilation is automatically resumed if the respiratory rate exceeds a preset value.

3. Capnography. This may be useful to detect periods of alveolar hypoventilation and hyperventilation (Fevrier et al. 1985).

4. CO_2-controlled ventilation. Chopin et al. (1983) described a weaning method called "CO_2 MV" in which the spontaneous or mechanical mode of ventilation was automatically determined by the level of the end-expiratory carbon dioxide concentration ($F_{ET}CO_2$). In the absence of acute cardiopulmonary complications, the gradient between the arterial ($PaCO_2$) and end-expiratory ($P_{ET}CO_2$) carbon dioxide partial pressures is assumed to be constant during the weaning process, so that an increase in $P_{ET}CO_2$ should indicate an increased $PaCo_2$. However, a decrease of $P_{ET}CO_2$ may be due to either acute circulatory failure or to significant tachypnea with augmentation of dead space ventilation. Schematically, three thresholds are preselected: a maximum threshold ($F_{ET}CO_2$ max), a minimum threshold ($F_{ET}CO_2$ min), and an intermediate threshold ($F_{ET}CO_2$ int). In the spontaneous mode of ventilation, $F_{ET}CO_2$ must lie between $F_{ET}CO_2$ min and $F_{ET}CO_2$ max (interval of spontaneous breathing). The spontaneous mode is allowed as long as $F_{ET}CO_2$ lies between these two thresholds. If $F_{ET}CO_2$ increases above $F_{ET}CO_2$ max or decreases below $F_{ET}CO_2$ min, the mechanical ventilation is automatically triggered so that the risk of alveolar hypoventilation is considerably reduced. In the controlled mode of ventilation, $F_{ET}CO_2$ lies between $F_{ET}CO_2$ min and $F_{ET}CO_2$ int (interval of controlled ventilation). The duration of the periods of mechanical ventilation is preselected and can range from 2 to 15 min, and beyond this preset duration, the spontaneous mode of ventilation is automatically resumed. Thus, a succession of periods of mechanical ventilation and spontaneous breathing may be observed.

5. Servocontrol of MMV Based on Capnography. Ben Ayed and Lemaire (1986) developed an algorhythm by which the preset V_E varies according to the expired CO_2. The increase of $P_{ET}CO_2$ triggers a rise of the preset V_E that can be achieved by increasing the rate of mechanical breaths (CPU1) or adding a pressure support (Veolar). A decrease of $P_{ET}CO_2$ induces a diminution of the preset V_E if the ventilatory mode is mainly mechanical or triggers IMV if the ventilatory mode is mainly spontaneous. This algorhythm has been tested in 17 patients, with especially good results when the rate of mechanical breaths was used to modify the preset V_E (Ben Ayed and Lemaire 1986).

The MMV may induce, as IMV, an excessive increase of the work of breathing resulting from the high resistance of the ventilator breathing system particularly the humidifier (Mecklenburgh et al. 1986) and the amount of negative pressure that the patient must generate to activate the demand valve (Cameron and Oh 1986).

The safety provided by the MMV system during spontaneous breathing may result in a diminution of supervision and physiotherapy care. Moreover, stimulation of the patient by the staff to breathe spontaneously may be less than during T-piece breathing.

Other complications are related to specific ventilators:

1. CPU1. It was argued that altering the frequency of mechanical breaths did not always fulfill the patient's needs. For instance, an increase in ventilatory demand to overcome CO_2 rebreathing may only be achieved by an increase in spontaneous breathing, leading to respiratory muscles fatigue. In this respect, the CPU1 MMV is mainly a safety system, protecting against a reduction of spontaneous breathing.
2. Veolar. When IPS is left uncontrolled, very high levels may be reached, leading to apnea and deleterious increase in intrathoracic pressures. Limitation of tidal volume size and/or IPS levels should be included in this mode for increased safety and patient tolerance.

Factors Influencing the Ventilatory Mode During MMV

Injection of Sedatives

Injection of sedative drugs which decrease the ventilatory drive inducing apnea or severe alveolar hypoventilation will automatically trigger mechanical ventilation.

MMV and Nutrition

We performed a study to determine if the ventilatory mode (spontaneous or mechanical) and the $PaCO_2$ in patients receiving ventilatory support with MMV were dependent on the nutritional intake (Laaban et al. 1985). Eight stable patients received during 24 h a different caloric intake: diet A (mean, 430 kcal/day), diet B (mean, 2400 kcal/day), and diet C (mean 3300 kcal/day). Each patient received the three regimens in a random order, the preset V_E remaining unchanged. The preset V_E (mean, 9 /mn) was arbitrarily defined as being equal to 75% of the minute ventilation that ensured during mechanical ventilation a $PaCO_2$ between 30 and 40 mmHg while the patient was receiving a stable caloric intake (mean, 2000 kcal/day during 1 week). A 24 h respiratory monitoring (Critikon 8500) was performed during each period and the percentage of spontaneous ventilation over 24 h was computed. CO_2 production ($\dot{V}CO_2$), O_2 consumption ($\dot{V}O_2$), and respiratory quotient were measured using the classical method of indirect calorimetry and arterial blood gas values were determined during each period of caloric intake. The percentage of spontaneous ventilation over 24 h increased markedly with caloric intake from 11% (diet A) to 50% (diet B) and 79% (diet C) and was closely related to the increase of $\dot{V}CO_2$ with caloric intake. $PaCO_2$ increased with caloric intake, from a mean value of 33 mmHg (diet A) to 37 mmHg (diet B) and 40 mmHg (diet C), but hypercapnia developed only in those patients with chronic obstructive lung disease, with

$PaCO_2$ ranging between 45 and 50 mmHg during the hypercaloric diet C. Thus, the patient's ventilatory mode under MMV is closely dependent on the nutritional intake, as an increase in the spontaneous breathing mode may be induced by a high caloric intake, provided other conditions are constant. This increment in spontaneous breathing is probably due to the increase in $\dot{V}CO_2$ induced by caloric intake.

Indications for MMV

MMV should not just be considered only as a method of weaning patients from mechanical ventilation, but as a mode of mechanical ventilatory support per se.

Indications for MMV as a Weaning Method

MMV appears to be an interesting weaning method for patients who have undergone general anesthesia for major surgery. The wakening period is characterized by spontaneous breathing. MMV allows opiates to be administered safely during the postoperative period: if respiratory depression occurs, the mechanical ventilation is automatically triggered. MMV may be very useful in the postoperative management of patients with myasthenia gravis (Higgs and Bevan 1979); if the respiratory muscle power deteriorates for any reason, the MMV system ensures the patient will receive the preset V_E.

In theory, MMV is not a suitable method for weaning patients with chronic obstructive lung disease (COLD) requiring ventilatory support for an acute exacerbation: the excessive increase in the work of breathing that may develop during the periods of spontaneous breathing could lead to respiratory muscle fatigue. However, Chopin et al. (1987) showed that CO_2-regulated ventilation (CO_2-MV) could be an efficient method to wean COLD patients from ventilatory support. Forty-two COLD patients with acute respiratory failure (ARF) needing mechanical ventilation were randomly assigned to one of three different weaning modes: T-piece, IMV, or CO_2-MV. The $PaCO_2$ was lower during the weaning period in the CO_2-MV group. The number of patients who could be successfully weaned from mechanical ventilation was higher in the CO_2-MV group (13/14) than in the T-piece group (10/14) and the IMV group (5/14).

Apart from this work, no study has yet been performed to determine whether MMV shortens the duration of the weaning process or whether it could be useful for weaning patients in whom the usual weaning methods have failed.

Indications of MMV as a Ventilatory Support Mode

The patients most likely to benefit from MMV are those needing protracted ventilatory support and not suffering from acute or chronic lung disease (Table 1). MMV appears to be especially indicated in the following conditions:

Table 1. Mandatory minute volume ventilation (MMV) for patients

Patient no.	Sex	Age (years)	Disease	Previous Ventilation Mode	Previous Ventilation Duration (days)	Weaning criteria P. insp max (cm H$_2$O)	Weaning criteria Resting min vent (l/min)	Outcome	MMV Initial	MMV Final	Duration (days)
1	F	59	Cerebral hemorrhage, stress ulcer, gastrectomy	IMV	37	−23	11	S, W	10	8	6
2	F	27	Guillain-Barré syndrome	CMV	75	−20	6	S	6.5	6.5	4
3	M	33	Acute pancreatitis	IMV	30	−40	12	S, W	12	13	8
4	F	74	Guillain-Barré syndrome	CMV	105	−23	12	S	7.5	9	8
5	F	26	Myopathy: diaphragmatic paralysis (VC = 21% of predicted)	CMV	30	−24	6.4	S	7	5.5	4
6	M	61	Pancreatitis	IMV	30	−30	9	S, W	12	12	10
7	M	52	Zollinger-Ellison syndrome, duodenal ulcer perforated into abdominal aorta, peritoneal abscess	CMV	30	−35	5.6	S	14	15	5
8	M	56	Cerebral hemorrhage	IMV	35	−40	12	S	5.5	6.5	5
9	F	37	Polymyositis	CMV IMV	60	−25	6	S	9	5	6
10	M	62	Endocarditis, cerebral embolism	CMV	8	−35	12	D	9.6	9.6	4

S, surviving; D, deceased; W, weaned; IMV, intermittent mandatory ventilation; CMV, controlled mechanical ventilation

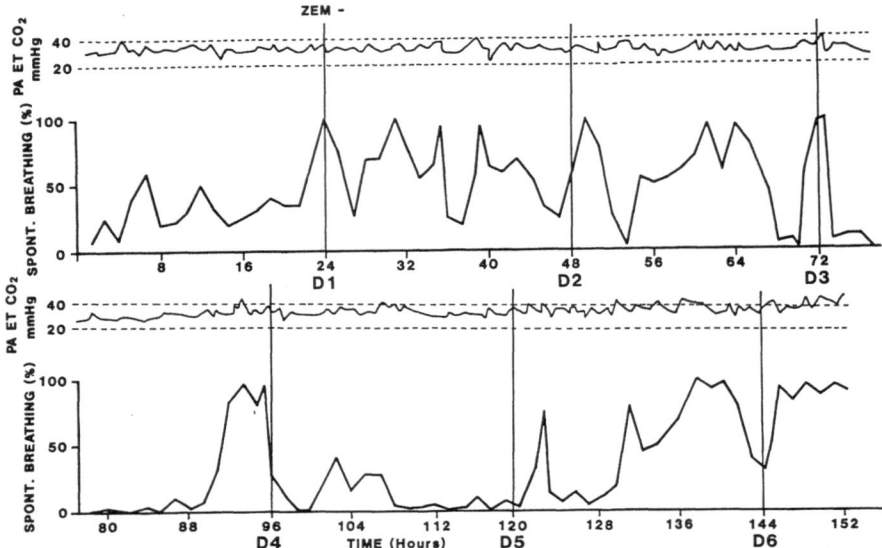

Fig. 6. A recording of $P_{ET}CO_2$ (upper trace) and the percentage of spontaneous ventilation (lower trace) for 6 days during an acute episode of polymyositis. $P_{ET}CO_2$ remained nearly constant during both spontaneous and mechanical ventilation. *Two dotted lines* represent the preset alarm limits of $P_{ET}CO_2$; *spont breathing*, percentage of spontaneous breathing

1. Complications of abdominal surgery (laparostomy, fistula, pancreatitis). MMV may prevent atrophy of the respiratory muscles and allows the safe administration of opiates before painful treatment. In the MMV mode, an increase in minute ventilation automatically matches any increase in the ventilatory needs (induced, for instance, by variations of nutritional intake).
2. Recovery from respiratory muscle paralysis due to neuro-muscular diseases (Guillain-Barré syndrome, myositis, myopathy, myasthenia gravis) (Fig. 6, 7).
3. Diseases with wide fluctuations of respiratory drive due to encephalopathy or repeated general anesthesia or intermittent use of sedative drugs.

Conversely, MMV should not be used in patients with increased work of breathing, or in acute pulmonary disease, or in the presence of decreased performance of the respiratory muscles.

In fact, only a few studies have assessed the value of MMV as a ventilatory support mode (Ben Ayed et al. 1985; Fevrier et al. 1985; Laaban et al. 1985). Fevrier et al. (1985) studied the efficiency and safety of MMV in ten non-COLD patients who needed a prolonged mechanical ventilation for complications of abdominal surgery $(n = 3)$, neurological disease $(n = 5)$, and muscular disease $(n = 2)$. MMV was provided by a CPU 1 ventilator and the monitoring of ventilatory parameters including expired CO_2 was performed using the

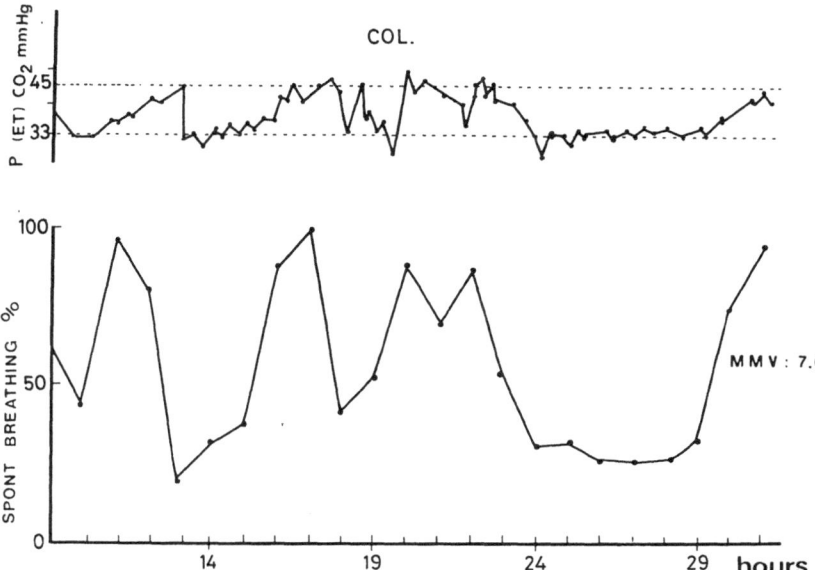

Fig. 7. A recording of $P_{ET}CO_2$ (upper trace) and the percentage of spontaneous breathing (lower trace) in a patient with Guillain-Barré syndrome. Several times each day, the patient increased her frequency of spontaneous breathing with small tidal volumes, but hypercapnia rapidly ensued causing the $P_{ET}CO_2$ to reach the upper alarm level. Without any staff intervention, mechanical cycles resumed, triggered by small tidal volumes lower than the minimal V_T

Ohmeda monitor. MMV was employed for a total of 46 days (mean duration of MMV for each patient, 5 ± 1.4 days) and no accident or incident was observed. Five patients were completely weaned off their ventilatory support at the end of the MMV study period. A few episodes of alveolar hypoventilation occurred that were detected by an increase of $P_{ET}CO_2$, but the $PaCO_2$ never exceeded 45–50 mmHg. Controlled ventilation was resumed in one patient with an intraperitoneal abcess who developed hyperventilation with a marked decrease of $PaCO_2$.

Conclusions

MMV is an original mode of ventilatory support in which spontaneous breaths are combined with mechanical breaths while the patient is guaranteed to receive a preset minute ventilation. Further studies are needed to demonstrate formally the clinical usefulness of this ventilatory mode and further improvements are likely to appear soon in this rapidly evolving field. Microcomputing and electronic control of all machine settings, available now on any recent ventilator, have started to promote active research in the field of servocontrol. The present modalities of MMV, that we are using now, will probably become the harbingers for more modern methods of mechanical ventilation.

References

Ben Ayed M, Lemaire F (1986) Asservissement de la ventilation imposée variable (VIV) á la capnographie ($P_{ET}CO_2$) (Abstr). Reanim Soins Intensive Med Urgence 2:261

Ben Ayed M, Axler O, Lemaire F (1986) Un accident de la ventilation avec aide inspiratoire: bradypnée avec hyperinsufflation thoracique (Abstr). Reanim Soins Intensive Med Urgence 2:262

Benzer H (1982) The value of intermittent mandatory ventilation. Intensive Care Med 8:267–268

Boyer F, Jay S, Gaussorgues P, Methani K, Robert D (1988a) A new approach to mandatory ventilation: pressure support mandatory minute frequency. Am Rev Respir Dis [Suppl] 137:A476

Boyer F, Methani K, Lassonery S, Durante G, Gaussorgues P, Piperno D, Robert D (1988b) Ventilations mécaniques partielles: libertés et contraintes. Reanim Soins Intensive Med Urgence 2:262

Cameron PD, Oh TE (1986) Newer modes of mechanical ventilatory support. Anaesth Intensive Care 14:258–266

Chopin C, Fourrier F, Chambrin MC, Mangalaboyi J, Durocher A, Dubois D, Zakhama B, Wattel F (1983) Nouvelle technique de sevrage de l'assistance ventilatoire: ventilation asservie au gaz carbonique. Presse Med 12(8):495–497

Chopin C, Lestavel P, Fourrier F, Chambrin MC, Mangalaboyi J (1987) Techniques de ventilation destinées au sevrage. Réanimation et Médecine d'Urgence. Expansion Scientifique Française, Paris, pp 45–46

Christopher KL, Good JT, Bowman JL, Eberle DJ, Irvin C, Neff TA (1981) Should COPD patients be weaned by T-piece or IMV? A comparison of pressure and resistance in different systems. Chest 80:381

Covelli HD, Black JW, Olsen MS, Beekman JF (1981) Respiratory failure precipitated by high carbohydrate loads. Ann Intern Med 95:579–581

Fevrier MJ, Pilorget A, Lemaire F (1985) Efficacité clinique de la ventilation imposée variable (VIV, en anglais: MMV). Intérêt de la surveillance par capnographie (Abstr). Reanim Soins Intensive Med Urgence 1:249

Gilston A (1977) Intermittent mandatory ventilation: are IMV, MMV, PEEP or sighing advantageous? Anaesthesia 32:665–667

Hewlett AM, Platt AS, Terry VG (1977) Mandatory minute volume: a new concept in weaning from mechanical ventilation. Anaesthesia 32:163–169

Higgs BD, Bevan JC (1979) Use of mandatory minute volume ventilation in the perioperative management of a patient with myasthenia. Br J Anaesth 51:1181–1183

Laaban JP, Lemaire F, Baron JF, Harf A, Trunet P, Bonnet JL, Teisseire B (1985) Caloric intake influences on the respiratory mode during mandatory minute volume (MMV) ventilation. Chest 87:67–72

Lemaire F, Rieuf P (1983) Ventilation assistée intermittente (IMV), ventilation imposée variable (MMV), aide inspiratoire. Réanimation et Médecine d'Urgence. Expansion Scientifique Française, Paris, pp 305–314

Mathru M, Rao TLK, Venus B (1983) Ventilator-induced barotrauma in controlled mechanical ventilation versus intermittent mandatory ventilation. Crit Care Med 11:359–361

Mecklenburgh JS, Latto IP, AL-Obaidi TAA, Swai EA, Mapleson WW (1986) Excessive work of breathing during intermittent mandatory ventilation. Br J Anaesth 58:1048–1054

Nunn JF, Lyle DJR (1986) Bench testing of the CPU1 ventilator. Br J Anaesth 58:653–662
Ravenscroft PJ (1978) Simple mandatory minute volume. Anaesthesia 33:246–249
Sonne LJ, Davis JA (1982) Increased exercise performance in patients with severe COPD following inspiratory resistive training. Chest 81:436–439
Weisman IM, Rinaldo JE, Rogers RM, Sanders MH (1983) Intermittent mandatory ventilation. Am Rev Respir Dis 127:641–647

Special Indications

Mechanical Ventilation in Anesthesia

J. Marty and Y. Nivoche

Mechanical ventilation is increasingly used during anesthesia. About 40% of patients undergoing general anesthesia were being ventilated during and after the procedure at the end of the 1970s (Hatton et al. 1983). Its use is one of the major factors implicated in the decrease of perioperative mortality over the past 25 years. Indeed, this technique allows surgical procedures to be performed which would have been impossible with spontaneous breathing. In addition, artificial ventilation ensures correct pulmonary gas exchange during surgery and anesthesia in patients with normal lungs and in patients with respiratory or cardiac failure by avoiding alterations of respiratory function associated with anesthesia. Mechanical ventilation, which is a simple technique in most anesthetized patients whose lungs are healthy, is the most widely used. It allows a long-term adequacy of ventilation in contrast to manual ventilation.

Mechanical Ventilation in Anesthesia: Why?

Artificial ventilation is used during anethesia to avoid or minimize alterations of respiratory function induced by anesthetic agents or surgical procedures. These changes are increased in patients with respiratory failure.

Modification of Respiratory Function During Anesthesia

Alveolar Hypoventilation General anesthetics depress the respiratory drive by a direct effect on the respiratory centers in the central nervous system. Volatile anesthetics induce a decrease of tidal volume without adequate compensation by an increase in respiratory rate (Pavlin 1981). This effect depends on alveolar concentrations of halogenated anesthetics. For instance, at the level of 1 MAC, during spontaneous ventilation, $PaCO_2$ increases up to 50 torr with halothane or isoflurane or 60 torr with enflurane (Pavlin 1981). In adults at the level of 1.5 MAC, $PaCO_2$ is usually above 60 torr with the 3 agents (Marshall and Wyche 1972). More severe hypercarbias are observed in newborn infants or in elderly patients. In addition, compensatory responses to increased or decreased $PaCO_2$ are reduced by halogenated anesthetics. Barbiturates and benzodiazepines also depress the respiratory drive with apnea at the time of induction followed by a decrease in tidal volume. Narcotic agents modify alveolar ventilation in several ways (Stanley 1981). First, they decrease the respiratory drive in a dose-dependent fashion with a reduction in respiratory response to hypercapnia. With small doses, a decrease in respiratory rate without alteration of tidal volume may occur. With higher doses, the tidal volume is reduced as well. Second, morphine or meperidine can produce alveolar hypoventilation as a result of bronchoconstriction. Third, with drugs such as fentanyl, alveolar hypoventilation can be related to a decrease in chest wall compliance resulting from muscle rigidity. Finally, spontaneous ventilation is compromised when large doses of i.v. anesthetics or high concentrations of volatile anesthetics are used. Obviously, curarization increases these alterations. The recent anesthetic protocols which consist of high doses of narcotics to lower stress responses to surgery, impose artificial ventilation whatever the surgical procedure.

The posture of the patient or the surgical procedure itself can be responsible for alveolar hypoventilation by decreasing the performance of the respiratory muscles and by increasing the work of breathing. These factors occur during laparotomy and thoracotomy. During celioscopy, both posture (Trendelenburg) and high intraabdominal pressures increase respiratory work.

Other mechanisms can lead to alveolar hypoventilation during anesthesia (Benumof 1986). Anesthetic circuits and one-way valves may markedly increase respiratory resistance. When using deliberate hypotension, there is an increase in alveolar dead space as a result of alveoli being ventilated but hypoperfused.

Alteration of Blood Gas Exchange. Two main factors are involved in these changes; (a) an increase in ventilation, perfusion mismatching (Dueck et al. 1980; Marsh et al. 1973); (b) a reduction in functional residual capacity (FRC) (Rounds and Brody 1984). The alveolar-arterial PO_2 gradient increases with the decrease in FRC. Once FRC becomes, at least in part, lower than closing volume, airway closure occurs and the arterial PO_2 begins to fall (Don et al. 1972). Consequently, low VA/Q areas are more numerous. This phenomenon is more marked (Benumof 1986) in the following situations: major decrease in FRC; FRC previously low; closing volume previously high. A 15%-20% reduction in FRC is usually observed just after induction of anesthesia. The maximal decrease is reached several minutes after loss of consciousness and remains at this level during anesthesia and during the early period of recovery. Recent studies using tomodensitometry or other new methods evaluating thoracoabdominal geometry have given more detailed knowledge of the mechanisms involved in these phenomena (Hedenstierna et al. 1985).

When patients are anesthetized in the supine position, the FRC is lowered by a cephalic shift of diaphragm and by a central redistribution of blood volume. The upward shift of diaphragm is more important when muscle relaxants are used (Marsh et al. 1973).

Anesthesia modifies the tone of the respiratory muscles (Freund et al. 1964). In the awake state, the end expiratory tone of the inspiratory muscles is equilibrated at FRC with elastic recoil of the lungs. Just after induction of anesthesia, the end expiratory tone of inspiratory muscles falls while sustained activity of expiratory muscles becomes apparent. The resulting increase in abdominal pressure pushes the diaphragm upwards and reduces FRC.

Alteration of the mucocilia system may be due to the following factors (Benumof 1986): (a) dry gas mixture, (b) insufficiently warmed gases, (c) high inspired concentration of oxygen (d) anesthetic agents themselves.

The surgical posture (Benumof 1986; Marsh et al. 1973) affects breathing. The supine position is associated with increased perfusion in the dependent parts of the lungs. All areas located below the left atrium are in zone 3 (low $\dot{V}A/\dot{Q}$ ratio). Fluid overload will decrease the FRC and increase the shunt by producing of interstitial edema in the dependent areas. The Trendelenburg position has a more marked effect than the supine position. During celioscopies, the insufflation of air exaggerates the hazardous situation. Most of the alveoli are below the left atrium (zone 3). Consequently, the Trendelenburg posture is poorly tolerated in patients with left ventricular failure or mitral stenosis. In the lateral position, the lower lung is in zone 3. The compliance and FRC of this lung are decreased.

The use of inspired oxygen concentrations higher than 21% avoids hypoxemia. However, high inspired oxygen concentration may increase the proportion of areas with very low $\dot{V}A/\dot{Q}$ ratio due to alveolar collapse. This phenomenon can be avoided, at least in part, by using a more insoluble gas such as nitrogen in an oxygen-air mixture instead of oxygen alone. Finally, to ensure adequate arterial oxygenation during anesthesia, at least 30% oxygen should be administered.

Other adverse factors may be involved, including:

1. The inhibition of hypoxic vasoconstriction increases venous admixture. This can be observed with vasodilators (Benumof 1986) or with halogenated anesthetics, even if it is disputed by some authors (Palvin 1981).
2. The geometry of the diaphragm may be altered by curarization. The lower part of the diaphragm is pushed upwards by the guts. The proportion of areas with low $\dot{V}A/\dot{Q}$ is increased (Benumof 1986; Rounds and Brody 1984).
3. Changes in cardiac output may worsen the consequences of an intrapulmonary shunt (Benumof 1986). When the cardiac output is reduced compared with the oxygen requirement ($\dot{V}O_2$), the oxygen content in the venous blood is reduced. As a consequence, the arterial blood which is a mixture of oxygenated blood and of shunted venous blood is further desaturated. Such a decrease in cardiac output may occur during or after surgery and anesthesia if associated with bleeding, hypovolemia, or heart failure.

Alteration of Respiratory Function During Recovery from Anesthesia

Several reasons can explain some of the postoperative respiratory disturbances excluding complications such as pulmonary aspiration, pulmonary edema, or atelectasis due to endobronchial intubations. The residual effects of anesthetic agents may account for the changes in the early period (Marshall and Wyche 1972). Obstruction with apnea may be observed, but more frequently hypoventilation occurs which has a complex time course. During surgery, nociceptive stimulation overrides the depressive effects of anesthetic agents on respiratory drive. When surgical stimulation stops, respiratory depression may appear. Another factor may be the recirculation of narcotics which can induce delayed respiratory depression. The decrease in FRC is still present during the early postoperative period and hypoxia can result. Circulatory and temperature changes may also be implicated in hypoxic states because of the associated venous oxygen desaturation. This phenomenon is observed when cardiac output is low (hypovolemia, cardiac failure) or when oxygen consumption is high (shivering). Surgical incision decreases the performance of the respiratory system in several ways: The vital capacity is reduced by 30% after upper abdominal surgery or thoracotomy; the pain of the incision impairs the evacuation of bronchial secretions (Benumof 1986) after upper abdominal surgery and diaphragmatic dysfunction may still be present 8 h after extubation. Finally, cooling of the phrenic nerves by ice may result in partial paralysis of the diaphragm.

Influence of Pulmonary Diseases

All the phenomena described above are worsened by preexisting respiratory diseases (Benumof 1986). For example, in chronic obstructive pulmonary disease (COPD) the closing volume is already increased, there is increased airway resistance, and there are areas of the lung with a low $\dot{V}A/\dot{Q}$ ratio. The risks of postoperative hypoxemia and hypoventilation are obviously increased under these circumstances. Heavy smokers also have a high closing volume, alterations of small airways, and $\dot{V}A/\dot{Q}$ mismatching. Obesity is associated with a decrease in FRC and patients with interstitial or alveolar diseases have preexisting hypoxemia with low FRC and $\dot{V}A/\dot{Q}$ mismatching.

Mechanical Ventilation: How?

Although mechanical ventilation during anesthesia and in the postoperative period is normally a simple process, all ventilators should comply with the current safety criteria.

Ventilators

Ventilation during anesthesia aims to avoid alveolar hypoventilation induced by anesthesia and surgery in patients with healthy lungs. The ventilator must be fitted with the standard safety devices and may be adapted to provide inhalation anesthesia.

Characteristics of the Ventilator. The ventilator may be designed to be stationed in the operating room alone or it may be constructed in modular form for mobile use outside the operating room. The *general characteristics* are:

1. The type of energy used does not matter.
2. The compliance and resistance of the patient-circuit system are continuously modified during anesthesia. These variations must not alter the characteristics of ventilation. The properties of the ideal ventilator have been reported elsewhere (Tremolieres 1983). Flow generators are best as the tidal volume will not change with change in the patient's lung characteristics.
3. Fully controlled mechanical ventilation is the main mode of ventilation for anesthesia with the occasional use of positive end expiratory pressure (PEEP). Other modes involve more complicated procedures for tuning and the evaluation of these modes of ventilation cannot be easily performed during anesthesia.
4. Tuning parameters. The following complementary characteristics are usual:

   —Tidal volume ranging from 7 to 15 ml/kg.
   —Inspiratory flow from 0.3 to 1 l/s.
   —Intermittent positive pressure ranging from 0 to 6 kPa.
   —Respiratory rate ranging from 0.1 to more than 1 Hz.
   —I/E ratio ranging from 1/3 to 1 rather than fixed at 1/2.

   the choice of values higher than 1 must be protected by mechanical or electronic devices.
5. Other materials are useful, like humidifiers and warmers; however, artificial noses are also efficient.

The following devices are necessary for safety:

1. Impossibility of delivering a gas mixture with less than 21% oxygen.
2. Oxygen bypass with an instantaneous flow above 35 l/min.
3. System for analysis of oxygen concentration, temperature of inspired gas, expiratory volumes, pressure of O_2, air and N_2O instantaneous and mean pressures in the circuits, concentration of inhalational agents, and carbon dioxide concentration.
4. Alarms signalling failure of power source, failure of O_2 supply, oxygen concentration (high and low value alarms), disconnection of patient from ventilator, expired minute volume (high and low value alarms), and overpressure in airways.

Compatibility with Anesthetic Techniques. Ventilation for anesthetized patients must take into account the problems associated with inhalation anesthesia. In addition, anesthetic agents may alter the reliability of monitoring devices. These problems are particularly important in children. The ventilator must allow the rapid shift from controlled ventilation to spontaneous breathing without altering the ability to monitor expiratory volume, whatever the kind of circuit used (open or closed). Scavanging devices must not modify the mechanics of the system.

The composition of the inspired gas mixture is determined upstream of the ventilator. In contrast, it is determined directly in the circuit when closed circuits are used. This implies that flowmeters are accurate for flows below 1 l/min. The performances of vaporizers are altered by changes in pressure, flow, or temperature.

The elastic properties of the pipes have an important effect on the real tidal volume delivered to the patient. A "squeezing" effect may be increased by the presence of humidifiers, filters, and measurement probes present in the circuit. For a given minute volume, the values of alveolar ventilation vary widely.

High flow rates and the use of one-way valves increase respiratory work. The use of N_2O is not systematic. Air-O_2 blenders allow ventilation of mixtures with inspired oxygen concentration below 60%.

Choice of ventilator. The choice of ventilator will be determined by the clinical requirement and by cost. Indeed, a single ventilator that can be used for open and closed systems, for adults and children, and for routine anesthesia as well as for long-term ventilation does not exist. High flows and one-way valves are used in the majority of cases. In anesthesia, a simple and cheap ventilator is sufficient (Adams and Henville 1977; Cazalaa et al. 1984; Ivanoff et al. 1977). When low flow, or Mapleson E circuits are used, the ventilator is very different (Bazaral 1981; Haberer and Schoeffler 1979; Kay et al. 1983). In 1989, there are a number of ventilators that are adequate for standard use in the operating room. The price ranges between 10 000 to 45 000 US dollars depending on the number of options available (many of them are not mandatory). In general, one-half the price is related to the cost of safety systems or vaporizers. More reliable and sophisticated ventilators with newly developed vaporization systems have appeared recently but the gains may be at the expense of simplicity. A high cost is questionable for routine anesthesia.

Ventilators for the recovery room are simpler since vaporizers and N_2O are not required. However, for some patients a more sophisticated ICU type ventilator may be required in the recovery room.

Management of Artificial Ventilation

The setting of the ventilator is relatively easy in the operating room since anesthetized patients tolerate mechanical ventilation without difficulty. Gas exchange requires a lower minute volume ventilation than in awake patients, since $\dot{V}O_2$ is reduced by anesthesia (Benhamou and Desmonts 1984). The aims of perioperative artificial ventilation are: (a) adjustment of alveolar ventilation to obtain an adequate $PaCO_2$; (b) maintenance of central temperature; (c) avoidance of complications.

Ventilation Modes. Intermittent positive pressure ventilation is the usual method. High tidal volumes with a relatively low respiratory rate are useful to avoid (A-a)PO$_2$ differences related to alveolar collapse (Primiano et al. 1982). Adjustment of ventilation according to the age of the patients is required as indicated in Table 1. If the minute volume is increased, the level of alveolar ventilation may be stabilized by increasing the dead space.

The use of PEEP has been proposed in anesthesia, but its efficiency has not been demonstrated (Rounds and Brody 1984). PEEP increases FRC and decreases the (A-a)PO$_2$ difference. However, PEEP during anesthesia: (a) has a less-predictable effect on PaO$_2$ than modificiation of inspired concentration of oxygen (Benumof 1984); (b) does not prevent late postoperative hypoxemia or ARDS (Rounds and Brody 1984); (c) increases the risk of paradoxical embolism. In contrast, its use may be interesting to lower the incidence of air embolism in neurosurgery. The presence of valves in circuits for children induces a degree of PEEP. Intermittent mechanical ventilation (IMV) and inspiratory pressure have been used to facilitate the return to spontaneous ventilation at the end of anesthesia. However, evaluation and management of these modes are difficult during anesthesia and they may induce unpredictable occlusion of the airways if the demand valves are too hard to trigger.

The closed system is more economical in the use of volatile anesthetics and gases. However, accurate adjustment of O$_2$ flow implies a need for analysis of the gases. The characteristics of the closed circuit allow easily controlled ventilation (Kofke and Latta 1982). Induction and recovery are performed with an open circuit.

High frequency ventilation is useful for some surgical procedures where immobility of the airways is required (larynx, lungs, mediastinum). However, the monitoring of tidal volume and humidification of the gas mixture are difficult.

Other Goals

Temperature. Ventilation with a dry and cool gas mixture is a major cause of hypothermia during anesthesia. The use of humidified and warmed gas allows the maintenance of body temperature. However, some risks are present, including (a) burns of upper airways at the beginning of ventilation may occur if the heater has been warmed up before ventilation is isolated and (b) an excess of water in airways. Artificial noses are a good alternative.

Prevention of Respiratory Infection. Humidification and heating of gas mixtures increase the risk of cross-infection. Circuits have to be decontaminated or disposable tubing is recommended. The growth of bacteria is uncommon during the first 24 h (Lareau et al. 1978). However, after ventilation of patients with infection or immunodeficiency, circuits must be changed or discarded. Bacteriological surveillance must be performed repeatedly.

Specific Techniques

Pediatric Anesthesia. The reliability of the respiratory parameters and monitoring devices is always altered. Tidal volume varies with modification of compliance or with leakage of gas. One-lung ventilation is difficult.

Endoscopy of Airways. Most ventilation modes have been used for these procedures. However, it is impossible to measure or predict the minute volume because of the important variations of resistance and of leakage. Overpressure in the airway is the main risk.

Monitoring and Mishaps of Artificial Ventilation

The principles of ventilation monitoring during anesthesia are different from those of ventilation in the ICU because patients are anesthetized and often paralyzed. The signs of an inadequate ventilation depend upon autonomic changes in heart rate and blood pressure or the development of cyanosis. The recording of these parameters should be performed frequently since the autonomy of these patients is very low. The complications of ventilation are the same as in other patients except the following.

Technical Hazards. Selective intubation is possible when the posture of the patient changes during the procedure. It leads to massive atelectasis and/or induces overpressure in the airways. Prevention of this accident consists of checking the respiratory parameters, ensuring the good function of both sides of the chest more by observation and auscultation, and double checking the position of the tracheal tube when the posture is changed.

Accidental disconnection of the patient from the ventilator and the inhalation of gas mixtures with an oxygen concentration below 21% are the most dramatic hazards of ventilation during anesthesia.

Alveolar Hyperventilation. This condition is frequently observed because anesthesia reduces the production of CO_2. Hyperventilation induces cellular hypoxia, lactic acidosis, circulatory failure, and hypothermia. It can delay recovery from anesthesia and produce an early postoperative hypoxemia. It is difficult to determine accurately the adequate level of ventilation during anesthesia without measuring the PCO_2 either in expiratory gases or in blood.

Hyperoxia. The hazards of perioperative hyperoxia are not well known because the exposure is time limited (Lamantia et al. 1984). The alteration of alveolar membranes and retina of newborns (Flynn 1984) younger than 45 weeks of gestational age are not correlated with anesthetic events. A prolonged hyperoxia may create alveolar collapse. However, the risks of hypoxia are greater than are the theoretical ones of hyperoxia.

Mechanical Ventilation During Anesthesia: When?

The indications for artificial ventilation are difficult to itemize. In addition, they differ markedly from one group to another particularly because of differences in operating procedures. However, some guidelines may be established. Mechanical ventilation is indicated in the following situations.

1. All surgical procedures which do not allow an efficient spontaneous ventilation as in thoracic surgery, cardiac surgery, upper abdominal surgery, or celioscopy.
2. Each surgical procedure which needs accurate control of blood gases; this is particularly important in neurosurgery.
3. Each anesthetic technique using muscle relaxants, high doses of narcotics, or a deep level of anesthesia. In these cases, spontaneous breathing is impossible.
4. Techniques which alter gas exchange such as deliberate hypotension, massive transfusion, or hemodilution. Other indications are more questionable.
5. Artificial ventilation is indicated when spontaneous breathing seems hazardous because the procedure lasts a long time. The risk is increased by several additional factors (hypothermia, immobility, dry secretions, alveolar hypoventilation, fatigue of respiratory muscles). The time limit varies with age, posture, or the surgical procedures. Mechanical ventilation is recommended if the procedure lasts longer than 60–90 min.
6. Patients with previous respiratory diseases are more frequently ventilated than others, particularly those with severe obstructive diseases. However, the need for ventilation cannot be predicted by preoperative functional evaluation.
7. Patients with cardiac disease. The indication is in fact frequently related to the use of high doses of narcotics except for short-term procedures.

The indications are more questionable during recovery except when postoperative respiratory complications are present.

The more common indication is related to residual effect of anesthesia particularly after the use of narcotics or muscle relaxants; it is generally short-term ventilation. The maintenance of ventilation during the postoperative period is frequently mandatory in patients with chronic or acute respiratory failure. After specific surgical procedures, such as lung, cardiac, or abdominal surgery, mechanical ventilation is not routinely indicated for postoperative ventilation; indeed, no controlled randomized trial, difficult to perform, has yet demonstrated the efficiency of this method. The same comment concerns patients with cardiac disease. Several groups have proposed postoperative ventilation with the maintenance of sedation to reduce paradoxical hemodynamic responses during recovery in order to reduce postoperative mortality; however, no controlled study has yet evaluated this approach.

References

Adams AP, Henville JD (1977) A new generation of anaesthetic ventilators. Anaesthesia 32:34–40
Bazaral MG (1981) Volume ventilation systems for infants. Anesthesiology 54:240–245
Bendixen HH, Hedley-Whyte D, Chir B, Laver MB (1963) Impaired oxygenation in surgical patients during general anesthesia with controlled ventilation. N Engle J Med 269:991–996

Benhamou D, Desmonts JM (1984) La consomation d'oxygène per et post-anesthésique. Ann Fr Anesth Reanim 3:205–211

Benumof JL (1984) Anesthesia for thoracic surgery. American Society of Anesthesiologist, New Orleans (Annual refresher course lectures, lecture 214)

Benumof JL (1986) Respiratory physiology and respiratory function during anesthesia. In: Miller RD (ed) Anesthesia, vol 2. Livingstone, New York, pp 1115–1164

Cazalaa JB, Louville Y, Weber B (1984) Respirateurs: fonctions et usages. Agressologie 25:2–4

Clergue F (1984) Le monitorage respiratoire per et post-opératoire. In: Desmonts JM (ed) Le monitorgage de l'opéré. Masson, Paris, pp 37–55 (Collection d'anesthésiologie et de réanimation chirurgicale et médicale vol 2)

Cooper JB, Newbower RS, Long CD, McPeek B (1978) Preventable anesthesia mishaps: a study of human factors. Anesthesiology 49:399–406

Cooper JB, Newbower RS, Welxh JP, Dedrick DF (1982a) Preparation for induction. In: Lebowitz PW, Newberg LA, Gillette MT (eds) Clinical anesthesia, 2nd edn. Little, Brown, Boston, (Procedures of the Massachusetts General Hospital), pp 10–40

Cooper JB, Long CD, Newbower RS, Philip JH (1982b) Critical incidents associated with intraoperative exchanges of anesthesia personnel. Anesthesiology 56:456–461

Cote CJ, Petkav AJ, Ryan JF, Welch JP (1983) Wasted ventilation measured in vitro with eight anesthetic circuits with and without inline humidification. Anesthesiology 59:442–446

De Vlieger H, Van Aede J, Van Hasebroeck P, Jaeken J, Eggermon E (1983) Diagram for easy volume setting of an infant ventilation. Crit Care Med 11:657–659

Don HF, Wahba WM, Craig DB (1972) Airway closure, gas trapping and the functional residual capacity during anesthesia. Anesthesiology 36:533–639

Dueck R, Young I, Clausen J, Wagner PD (1980) Altered distribution of pulmonary ventilation and blood flow following induction of inhalation anesthesia. Anesthesiology 52:113–125

Dureuil B, Desmonts JM, Mankikian B, Prokocimer P (1985) Effects of aminophyline on diaphragmatic dysfunction after upper abdominal surgery. Anesthesiology 62:242–246

Fisher DM (1983) Anesthesia equipment for pediatrics. In: Gregory GA (ed) Pediatric anesthesia, vol 1. Livingstone, Edinburgh, pp 347–380

Flynn JT (1984) Oxygen and retrolental fibroplasia: update and challenge. Anesthesiology 60:397–399

Freund F, Roos A, Dood RB (1964) Expiratory activity of the abdominal muscles in man during general anesthesia. J Appl Physiol 16:693–702

Haberer JP, Schoeffler P (1979) Les sytèmes semi-fermés dérivés du tube en T d'Ayre. Cah Anesthesiol 27:633–648

Hatton F, Tiret L, Maujol L, N'doye P, Vourc'h G, Desmonts JM, Otteni JC, Scherpereel P (1983) Inserm: Enquête épidémiologique sur les anesthésies. Ann Fr Anesth Reanim 2:333–365

Hedenstierna G, Strandberg A, Brismar R, Lundquist H, Syensson L, Tokics L (1985) Functional residual capacity, thoracoabdominal dimensions and central blood volume during general anesthesia with muscle paralysis and mechanical ventilation. Anesthesiology 62:247–254

Ivanoff S, Cazalaa JB, Weber B (1977) Respirateurs: caractères et fonctions. Agressologie 18:1–124

Kay B, Beatty PCW, Healy TEJ, Alloush MEA, Calpin YM (1983) Change in the work of breathing imposed by five anaesthetic breathing systems. Br J Anaesth 55:1239–1247

Kofke WA, Latta WB (1982) Closed circuit anesthesia. In: Lebowitz PW, Newberg LA, Gillette MT (eds) Clinical anesthesia, 2nd edn. Little, Brown, Boston, (Procedures of the Massachusetts General Hospital), pp 464–476

Lamantia KR, Glick JH, Marshall BE (1984) Supplemental oxygen does not cause respiratory failure in bleomycin-treated surgical patients. Anesthesiology 60:65–67

Lareau SC, Ryan KJ, Diener CF (1978) The relationship between frequency of ventilator circuit changes and injections hazard. Am Rev Respir Dis 118:493–496

Marsh HM, Rehder K, Sessler AD, Fowler WS (1973) Effects of mechanical ventilation muscle paralysis and posture on ventilation-perfusion relationship in anesthetized man. Anesthesiology 38:59–67

Marshall BE, Wyche MQ (1972) Hypoxemia during and after anesthesia. Anesthesiology 37:178–301

Pavlin EG (1981) Respiratory pharmacology of inhaled anesthetic agents. In: Miller RD, Anesthesia, vol 1. Churchill Livingstone, New York, pp 349–382

Primiano FP, Chatburn RL, Lough MD (1982) Mean airway pressure: theoretical considerations. Crit Care Med 10:378–383

Rounds S, Brody JS (1984) Putting PEEP in perspective. N Engl J Med 311:323–325

Stanley TH (1981) Pharmacology of intravenous narcotic anesthetics. In: Miller RD, Anesthesia, vol 1. Churchill Livingstone, New York, pp 425–449

Trémolières F (1983) Choix d'un respirateur. In: Réanimation et Médecine d'Urgence. Expansion Scientifique Française, Paris, pp 255–334

Ventilation in Thoracic Surgery

F. Bonnet, O. Boico, and M. Fischler

Thoracic surgery is commonly carried out in the lateral decubitus position and requires one-lung ventilation. These conditions impair the normal pattern of ventilation and pulmonary perfusion. These changes are responsible for the development of low $\dot{V}/\dot{Q}$ regions and/or true shunt. In some patients, these changes can lead to hypoxemia in spite of a higher oxygen concentration in the inspired gases. Several techniques of ventilation have been developed to improve gas exchange under these circumstances while at the same time also taking into account the needs of the surgeon.

Changes in Ventilation and Perfusion Due to Thoracic Surgery

Physiology of the Lateral Decubitus Position (LDP)

Awake, Closed Chest. Gravity causes a gradient in pleural pressure in LDP (Agostini 1972) such that the functional residual capacity (FRC) of the lower lung is inferior to that of the upper lung (Kaneko et al. 1966). In LDP, the dome of the lower diaphragm is pushed upwards by the weight of the abdominal contents and so lies higher than the dome of the upper diaphragm, as a result the lower diaphragm is more sharply curved and so it is able to contract more efficiently during spontaneous respiration (Roussos et al. 1977).

The alveoli of the lower lung have less volume at the end of expiration. They are thus located on a steeper part of the slope of the pressure-volume curve, and their compliance is higher than that of the alveoli of the upper lung. For the same variation in pleural pressure, the alveolar volume depends on regional compliance; it is therefore higher for the lower lung. Thus, in spontaneous respiration and in LDP, the lower lung receives most of the tidal volume (Kaneko et al. 1966).

Pulmonary perfusion follows a pressure gradient. In LDP, the lower lung is the better perfused. In the awake patient in LDP, the lower lung receives most of the ventilation and perfusion, so that the distribution of ventilation-perfusion ratios are relatively balanced (Rheder et al. 1979).

Anesthetized Patient. Thoracic surgery is carried out under controlled ventilation usually with the aid of muscular relaxation. Under these conditions the diaphragm does not contract (Rheder et al. 1972). The force set up by abdominal organs is more difficult to overcome in the lower regions (Chevrolet et al. 1978). In addition the weight of the mediastinum exerts itself on the lower lung (Froese and Bryan 1974). Thus, under controlled ventilation, the upper lung receives most of the tidal volume (Chevrolet et al. 1978; Rheder and Sessler 1973). Thoracotomy further emphasizes this phenomenon (Nunn 1961; Werner et al. 1984). The dependent lung continues to receive most of the pulmonary perfusion. Opening the chest causes a mismatching of ventilation with perfusion. The upper lung receives most of the ventilation and less perfusion and so it is the site of high ventilation-perfusion rates. The dependent lung receives most of the perfusion and less ventilation and so it is responsible for low VA/Q regions (Chevrolet et al. 1978; Rheder et al. 1979). In the most dependent part of the lower lung, perfusion pressure of the pulmonary vessels can be higher than intraalveolar pressure, thus creating the conditions for the development of atelectasis, responsible for the pulmonary shunt. Exclusion of the upper lung shifts the totality of ventilation towards the lower lung, thus creating a transpulmonary shunt. The importance of this shunt is limited by the changes in the distribution of perfusion. On the one hand, gravity restricts the perfusion of the upper lung, as discussed before. On the other hand, the decrease in oxygen alveolar tension (PaO_2) in the collapsed lung causes pulmonary vasoconstriction. Hypoxic pulmonary vasoconstriction (HPV) is responsible for an increase in vascular resistance in the collapsed lung. The consequence is a fall in the perfusion of that lung, and this prevails over the development of an important transpulmonary shunt (Benumof 1979).

The severity of the shunt induced by the collapse of the upper lung depends on the state of the preexisting parenchyma and the degree of HPV. If a pathological lung is operated upon or is already isolated for ventilation and perfusion, its exclusion during the surgical procedure has a minimal effect on gas exchange. HPV can be modified by different mechanical and pharmacological factors. In patients with chronic obstructive pulmonary disease (COPD) not only is the reactivity of the vascular bed diminished but HPV is blunted by a rise in pulmonary arterial pressure and hypocapnia (Benumof and Wahrenbrock 1975, 1977). It also depends on the mixed venous oxygen tension ($P\bar{v}O_2$), which when lowered induces a rise in HPV. If the shunt induced by the collapse of the upper lung is considerable, it can be responsible for hypoxemia and significant decrease in $P\bar{v}O_2$. This fall of the $P\bar{v}O_2$ in the lower, ventilated and perfused lung can provoke vasoconstriction and thus a redistribution of perfusion towards the upper lung, leading to a higher shunt (Benumof et al. 1981; Pease et al. 1982; Zasslow et al. 1982). The $P\bar{v}O_2$ can also be diminished by a perioperative decrease in the cardiac output. Laboratory experiments have shown that inhalational anesthetics decrease HPV (Biertnaes 1977; Matrhes et al. 1977; Pavlin et al. 1985; Pavlin and Winn 1986). In contrast, human studies suggest that, under the conditions of thoracic surgery, the use of inhalational anesthetics does not worsen the pulmonary shunt or hypoxemia (Carlsson et al. 1987; Rogers and Benumof 1985). Surgical maneuvers inhibit HPV by liberating vasodilating prostaglandins (Anderson and Benumof 1981; Piper and Vane 1971). On the other hand, lung collapse itself does not change corresponding perfusion.

Effects on Gas Exchange. It is possible to maintain a normocapnic status if one-lung ventilation is identical to the preoperative period (Bachand et al. 1975; Hatch 1966; Kerr 1972).

The appearance or worsening of low $\dot{V}/\dot{Q}$ regions or true shunt may be responsible for severe hypoxemia in some patients even when ventilated with an FiO_2 of 1 (100% oxygen). It is quite impossible to predict perioperative hypoxemia for a given patient even when a preoperative evaluation of ventilation and perfusion of each lung allows evaluation of the whole mechanism (Hurford et al. 1986; Katz et al. 1982). Hypoxemia is a more frequent finding in nonpulmonary thoracic surgery. After isolation of one lung, there is a gradual decrease in arterial oxygen tension (PaO_2) because of persisting diffusion of oxygen into the nonventilated lung (Katz et al. 1982). Hemodynamic changes are able to decrease the PaO_2 even when ventilation is stable (Fiser et al. 1982). Under these conditions, the monitoring of gas exchange by intermittent arterial blood gas analysis may be insufficient to detect hypoxemia in some patients. It is safer to use permanent monitoring. Transcutaneous PaO_2 is not always reliable in adults (Rithalia and Booth 1985; Rooth et al. 1976) and continuous and noninvasive monitoring of arterial oxygen saturation by pulse oxymetry is the most appropriate in these patients.

One-Lung Anesthesia Intubation

There are absolute and relative indications for separating the two lungs during operations or procedures. Isolation of one lung from the other is absolutely necessary:

1. In order to prevent spillage or contamination from an infected or bleeding lung to the noninvolved lung.
2. In case of large bronchopleural fistula or emphysematous cysts.

Separation of the lungs is relatively indicated when the collapse of one lung confers a critical benefit to the performance of surgery by facilitating surgical exposure; that is the case for repair of thoracic aortic aneurysm, upper lobectomy, and pneumonectomy.

Indications for the separation of the two lungs for other surgical procedures such as esophageal resection are less firm. There are several types of double-lumen endotracheal tubes (Carlens, White, Robertshaw, Bryce-Smith). In practice, the tip of the tube should be placed opposite the operated lung. The choice of the type of tube depends upon personal experience. A left sided tube is convenient for most cases requiring one-lung ventilation; if it is necessary to clamp the left mainstem bronchus, the tube can be withdrawn at that time into the trachea and then used in the same manner as a single-lumen endotracheal tube.

The tube is placed blindly into the appropriate bronchus, and the correct position is determined by:

1. A combination of unilateral clamping and unclamping with auscultation of the lungs.

2. Control of ventilation by spirometry of the two lungs and of each lung after clamping of the opposite one. The tube is malpositioned if one-lung ventilation is not identical with the two-lungs ventilation. The second method used to check the correct position of the tube is to confirm the absence of spirometry on the clamped side or the absence of bubbles when the free end of the clamped side is submerged in a beaker of water.
3. Fiberoptic bronchoscopy through the right lumen assessing the correct position of the tube in relation to the carina. The exact position of a double-lumen endotracheal tube has to be confirmed again after turning the patient to the lateral decubitus position.

Improvement of Gas Exchange

One-lung ventilation incurs a high risk of systemic hypoxemia. Thus, it is extremely important to maintain for as long as possible ventilation of the two lungs.

In most cases, increasing the inspired oxygen concentration over 70% allows correction of the decrease in PaO_2 due to isolation of one lung (Kerr 1972; Khanom and Branthwaite 1973; Tarhan and Lundborg 1970; Torda et al. 1974). Ventilation with $FiO_2 > 70\%$ must be initiated before isolation of one lung in order to increase residual oxygen in the separated lung. This step proportionally delays the decrease in PaO_2 after lung isolation.

In the small number of patients who develop a significant transpulmonary shunt and a PaO_2 less than 100 mmHg after collapse of the upper lung, gas exchange can be improved by applying a constant, positive pressure of 5–10 cm H_2O to the nonventilated lung (Alfery et al. 1981; Capan et al. 1980). This technique maintains in the non-ventilated lung a volume of oxygen depending on pulmonary compliance, which participates in gas exchange by diffusion.

Several very simple devices have been used to allow insufflation of the nondependent lung (Capan et al. 1980; Hannenber et al. 1984; Thiagarajah et al. 1984). Practically, it is enough to use an oxygen flowmeter with a reservoir bag provided with a safety valve and a manometer.

Persistent immobility of the insufflated lung insures good surgical conditions. Insufflation of oxygen at zero airway pressure is inefficient. A positive pressure of more than 15 cm H_2O is deleterious since it does not improve gas exchange and is responsible for an excessive inflation of the lung (Alfery et al. 1981). In theory, application of positive and expiratory pressure (PEEP) to the dependent ventilated lung allows increase in its FRC. The increase in FRC helps to prevent atelectasis (Brown et al. 1977; Rheder et al. 1973). But, in fact, the increase in the volume of the lower lung can cause compression of intraalveolar vessels responsible for an increase in pulmonary vascular resistance and the diversion of blood flow away from the ventilated to the non-ventilated lung (Benumof et al. 1979; Finley et al. 1963).

On the other hand, excessively high levels of PEEP may be responsible for a decrease in cardiac output and in PvO_2, thus contributing to a fall in the PaO_2 (Katz et al. 1982). There is strong advice against the very first use of PEEP on the lower lung. Association of PEEP on the lower lung to the insufflation of the upper lung does not provide any additional benefit (Alfery et al. 1981).

High-frequency ventilation (HPV) may be an interesting technique when there are hemodynamic problems together with ventilatory problems (Hildebrand et al. 1984). With HFV, intratracheal and pleural pressures are lower and cardiac output higher, while the transpulmonary shunt stays lower and PaO_2 higher than in traditional lung separation techniques of ventilation (El Baz et al. 1982; Malina et al. 1981). Thoracic aortic surgery would be an example of the potential application of this type of ventilation.

References

Agostini E (1972) Mechanics of the pleural space. Physiol Rev 52:57–128

Alfery DD, Benumof JL, Trousdale FR (1981) Improving oxygenation during one lung ventilation: the effects of PEEP and blood flow restriction to nonventilated lung. Anesthesiology 55:381

Anderson HW, Benumof JL (1981) Intrapulmonary shunting during one-lung ventilation and surgical manipulation. Anesthesiology 55:A377

Bachand R, Audet J, Meloche R, et al. (1975) Physiological changes associated with unilateral pulmonary ventilation during operations on one lung. Can Anaesth Soc J 22:659

Barker S, Tremper K (1986) A clinical comparison of transcutaneous PO_2 and pulse oximetry in the operating room. Anesth Analg 65:805–880

Benumof JL, Wahrenbrock EA (1975) Blunted hypoxic pulmonary vasoconstriction by increased lung vascular pressure. J Appl Physiol 38:846–850

Benumof JL, Wahrenbrock EA (1977) Dependency of hypoxic pulmonary vasoconstriction on temperature. J Appl Physiol 42:56–58

Benumof JL (1979) Mechanism of decreased blood flow to atelectatic lung. J Appl Physiol 46:1047–1048

Benumof JL, Rogers SN, Moyce PR, et al. (1979) Hypoxic pulmonary vasoconstriction and whole lung PEEP in the dog. Anesthesiology 51:503

Benumof JL, Pirlo AF, Johanson I, Trousdale F (1981) Interaction of PvO_2 on hypoxic pulmonary vasoconstriction. J Appl Physiol 51:871–874

Bjertnaes LJ (1977) Hypoxia induced vasoconstriction in isolated perfused lungs exposed to injectable or inhalation anesthetics. Acta Anaesthesiol Scand 21:133–147

Brown DR, Kafer ER, Roberson VO, et al. (1977) Improved oxygenation during thoracotomy with selective PEEP to the dependent lung. Anesth Analg 56:26

Capan LM, Turndorf H, Chandrakant P, et al. (1980) Optimization of arterial oxygenation during one lung anesthesia. Anesth Analg 59:847

Carlsson AJ, Hedenstierna G, Bindslev L (1987) Hypoxia induced vasoconstriction in human lung exposed to enflurane anaesthesia. Acta Anaesthesiol Scand 31:57–62

Chevrolet JC, Martin JG, Flood R, Martin RR, Engel LA (1978) Topographical ventilation and perfusion distribution during IPPB in the lateral posture Am Rev Respir Dis 118:847–854

El Baz NM, Kittle CF, Faber LP, Welsher W (1982) High frequency ventilation with an uncuffed endobronchial tube. J Thorac Cardiovasc Surg 84:823–828

Finley T, Hill TR, Bonica JJ (1963) Effect of intrapleural pressure on pulmonary shunt through atelectatic dog lung. Am J Physiol 205:1187

Fiser WP, Friday CD, Read RC (1982) Changes in arterial oxygenation and pulmonary shunt during thoracotomy with endobronchial anesthesia. J Thorac Cardiovasc Surg 83:523–531

Froese AB, Bryan CA (1974) Effects of anesthesia and paralysis on diaphragmatic mechanics in man. Anesthesiology 41:242–255

Hannenber AA, Sapwicz PR, Eienes RS, Jr, et al. (1984) A device for applying CPAP to the nonventilated upper lung during one lung ventilation. II. Anesthesiology 60:254

Hatch D (1966) Ventilation and arterial oxygenation during thoracic surgery. Thorax 21:310

Hildebrand PJ, Prakash D, Cosgrove J, Wilson JJ, Coppel DL (1984) High frequency jet ventilation. A method for thoracic surgery. Anaesthesia 39:1091–1095

Hurford WE, Kolfer AC, Strauss HW (1986) Use of ventilation/perfusion lung scans to predict oxygenation during one lung anesthesia. Anesthesiology 65:A479

Kaneko K, Milic Emili J, Dolovich MB, Dawsana M, Bates DV (1966) Regional distribution of ventilation and perfusion as a function of body position. J. Appl Physical 21 (7): 67–77

Katz JA, Laverne RG, Fairley HB, Thomas AN (1982) Pulmonary oxygen exchange during endobronchial anesthesia. Anesthesiology 56:164–171

Kerr JH (1972) Physiological aspects on one-lung (endobronchial) anesthesia. Int Anesthesiol Clin 10:61

Khanom T, Branthwaite MA (1973) Arterial oxygenation during one-lung anesthesia. I. A study in man. Anesthesia 28:132

Malina JR, Nordstrom SG, Sjostrand VH, Wattwil LM (1981) Clinical evaluation of high frequency positive pressure ventilation (HFPPV) in patients scheduled for open chest surgery. Anesth Analg 60:324–330

Mathers J, Benumof JL, Wahrenbrock EA (1977) General anesthetics and regional hypoxic pulmonary vasoconstriction. Anesthesiology 46:111–114

Miller FL, Malmkvist G, Cen L, Marshall C, Marshall BE (1985) Mechanical factors do not influence blood flow distribution in atelectasis. Anesthesiology 63:A522

Nunn JF (1961) The distribution of inspired gas during thoracic surgery. Ann R Coll Surg Engl 28:223

Pavlin EG, Reed RL, Winn RK (1985) Pulmonary vascular pressure-flow curves in intact goats demonstrate hypoxic pulmonary vasoconstriction is abolished by halothane. Anesthesiology 63:A532

Pavlin EG Winn RK (1986) Pulmonary vascular pressure-flow curves show hypoxic pulmonary vasoconstriction (HPV) is attenuated by isoflurane but not by thiamylal. Anesthesiology 65:A275

Pease RD, Benumof JL, Trousdale FR (1982) PAO_2 and pVO_2 interaction on hypoxic pulmonary vasoconstriction. J Appl Physiol 53:134–139

Piper P, Vane J (1971) The release of prostaglandins from lung and other tissues. Ann NY Acad Sci 180:363

Rheder K, Hatch DJ, Sessler AD, Fowler WS (1972) The function of each lung of anesthetized and paralyzed man during mechanical ventilation. Anesthesiology 37: 16–26

Rheder K, Sessler AD (1973) Function of each lung in spontaneously breathing man anesthetized with thiopental-meperidine. Anesthesiology 38:320–327

Rheder K, Wenthe FM, Sessler AD (1973) Function of each lung during mechanical ventilation with ZEEP and with PEEP in man anesthetized with thiopental-meperidine. Anesthesiology 39:597

Rheder K, Knopp TJ, Sessler AD, Didier P (1979) Ventilation-perfusion relationship in young healthy awake and anesthetized paralyzed man. J Appl Physiol 47:745–753

Rithalia S, Booth S (1985) Factors influencing transcutaneous oxygen tension. Intensive Care World 2:126–131

Rogers S, Benumof JL (1985) Halothane and isoflurane do not decrease paO_2 during one lung ventilation in intravenously anesthetized patients. Anesth Analg 64:946–954

Rooth G, Hedstrand V, Tyden H, Ogren C (1976) The validity of transcutaneous oxygen tension method in adults. Crit Care Med 4:162–165

Roussos CS, Martin RR, Engel LA (1977) Diaphragmatic contraction and the gradient of alveolar expansion in the lateral posture. J Appl Physiol 43:32

Tarhan S, Lundborg RO (1970) Effects of increased expiratory pressure on blood gas tensions and pulmonary shunting during thoracotomy with use of the Carlens catheter. Can Anaesth Soc J 17:4

Thiagarajah S, Job C, Rao A (1984) A device for applying CPAP to the nonventilated upper lung during one lung ventilation. I. Anesthesiology 60:253

Torda TA, McCulloch CH, O'Brien HD, et al. (1974) Pulmonary venous admixture during one-lung anesthesia: the effect of inhaled oxygen tension and respiration rate. Anaesthesia 29:272

Werner O, Malmkvist G, Beckman A, Stahle S, Nordstrom L (1984) Gas exchange and haemodynamics during thoracotomy. Br J Anaesth 56:1343–1349

Yelderman M, New W (1983) Evaluation of pulse oximetry. Anesthesiology 59:349–352

Zasslow MA, Benumof JL, Trousdale FR (1982) Hypoxic pulmonary vasoconstriction and the size of hypoxic compartment. J Appl Physiol 53:626–630

Independent Lung Ventilation

G. Conti, A. Pilorget and G. Crimi[1]

Independent lung ventilation (ILV) is a technique of respiratory support which may offer benefits in situations where conventional mechanical ventilation fails to manage certain patients with acute respiratory failure. Clinical reports concerning this elegant technique have steadily increased in recent years with the development of more biocompatible double lumen endobronchial tubes with high volume, low pressure cuffs.

As yet, however, no more than 70 cases of ILV have been published worldwide; moreover, no randomized trial exists comparing ILV with an alternative technique used in the treatment of unilateral acute lung injury: the lateral decubitus posture. It is therefore difficult to overcome the "case report philosophy" when dealing with ILV.

The aim of this chapter is to assess the present state of ILV. It will review the clinical conditions to be treated, the technical modalities of ILV, risks and possible complications, and finally it will analyze briefly the data emerging from the literature.

Indications

Unilateral Acute Lung Injury

Unilateral acute lung injury (ALI) is the result of a pathological process that involves one lung leaving the other unaffected. The inflammatory reactions in the diseased parenchyma lead to interstitial edema, loss of air space, and decreased compliance—all conditions separating the lungs into two units with totally different functional characteristics.

In the early stages of the syndrome, the preferential ventilation of the healthy lung does not give rise to gross $\dot{V}A/\dot{Q}$ mismatching due to the compensatory mechanisms producing a significant increase in the vascular resistance of the affected side (Benumof 1978; Fishman 1976). Thus, the injured lung is both hypoventilated and hypoperfused, while the other receives the bulk of both ventilation and perfusion (Fig. 1A). As a result, the overall $\dot{V}A/\dot{Q}$ matching is maintained within normal limits, which explains why, in the early stages of

---

[1] In memoriam

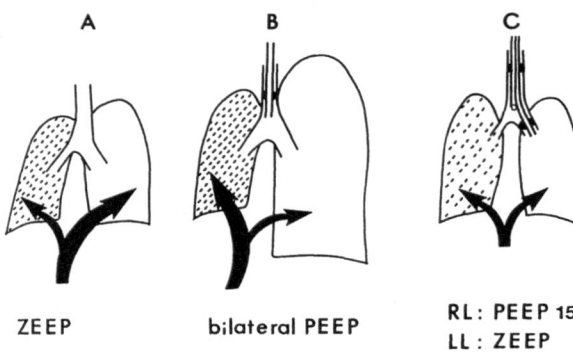

Fig. 1. **A** Ventilation and perfusion (black arrow) go to the normal lung. **B** Bilateral positive and expiratory pressure (PEEP) overdistends the normal lungs and redistributes perfusion to the diseased lung: $\dot{V}/\dot{Q}$ inhomogeneity is further increased. **C** Unilateral PEEP reexpands the diseased lung and equilibrates $\dot{V}$ and $\dot{Q}$ of each lung. ZEEP, zero end expiratory pressure

unilateral ALI, small increases in the inspired oxygen fraction are often sufficient to obtain satisfactory PaO_2 values. In a great number of patients, however, this situation is transient, and the compensatory mechanisms fail progressively, leading to hypoxemia.

Concurrent muscle fatigue often causes alveolar hypoventilation. At this stage, ventilatory support must be provided, and the patients may need to be connected to a source of intermittent or continuous positive pressure mechanical support. This treatment, however, can be inadequate, because of differences in the mechanical properties of the two lungs and preferential distribution of the tidal volumes of the less compliant resistant parenchyma. Alveolar hyperinflation and an increase of pulmonary vascular resistance results in shunting of blood to the diseased lung. As a result $\dot{V}A/\dot{Q}$ mismatching worsens with an increase of both "dead space" and "shunt-like" effects. If positive end expiratory pressure (PEEP) is applied or increased, the situation may further deteriorate because PEEP is preferentially transmitted to zones with more favorable time-constant values (Fig. 1B; Carlon et al. 1978a). In this situation, it is inappropriate to treat the lungs as if they were functionally similar, as they were now split by the pathological process into two units with totally different mechanical properties.

Bearing this concept in mind, two different approaches may be undertaken:

1. The reduction of the interpulmonary functional gradient
2. The separation of the two lungs followed by independent lung ventilation (Fig. 1C)

The first approach is achieved by the lateral decubitus position with the healthy lung in the dependent position. This is a relatively simple maneuver and should always be performed first as it is frequently effective. However, when it can not be employed or when it fails to manage the interpulmonary dyshomogeneity, ILV should be immediately employed with the modalities that are described below.

Bilateral Acute Lung Injury

Studies using computer tomography (CT) have shown that in most instances of diffuse parenchymal injury, the lungs are not homogeneously affected, the dependent lung regions being more collapsed than the nondependent. The resulting increase in $\dot{V}A/\dot{Q}$ mismatching is rarely modified by positive pressure ventilation, as this distributes tidal volumes and PEEP to the more compliant, nondependent zones of the lung.

A possible solution to this difficult problem has been proposed recently by Hedenstierna et al. (1984), who employed a combination of the lateral decubitus position with ILV. By turning the patient onto his side, the gravitational collapse of the parenchyma is be confined to the dependent lung while at the same time a net gain of functional residual capacity (FRC) is obtained in the nondependent lung. With separation of the lungs by means of a double-lumen tube, the dependent lung can be treated with adequate levels of PEEP, while ventilation can be selectively distributed to obtain a better ventilation/perfusion match.

This particular technique has proved to be successful both experimentally and in a limited number of patients (Bachrendtz and Hedenstierna 1984). Although interesting, this approach to bilateral ALI needs further clinical evidence to assess its efficacy. For this reason the following discussion about ILV will only address unilateral ALI.

Technical Modalities for ILV

Selection of Double-Lumen Tubes

The original Carlen's tubes were employed in the first reports of ILV for unilateral ALI, but it was soon clear that materials other than red rubber and a different shape were mandatory for long-term use as the presence of the carina "hook" could cause ulceration of the tracheal mucosa, and the lateral pressure transmitted to the tracheobronchial walls by the low compliant cuffs could induce ischemic lesions. The rigid nature of these tubes could cause damage to the upper airways, while the small diameter of the lumens makes tracheobronchial suction very difficult.

For all these reasons, the biluminal tubes now available for longterm use are manufactured with more histocompatible material (PVC), more compliant cuffs, an optional carina hook, and a lumen-to-wall ratio as high as possible. In addition, their pliability is a significant factor in patient comfort (Fig. 2).

More recently, a type of biluminal tube inserted via the tracheostomy tract has been tested; for the same internal diameter, it offers less resistance to

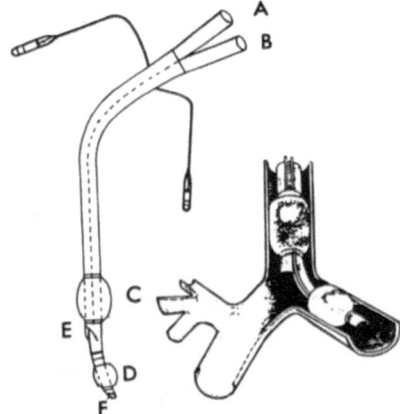

Fig. 2. Tracheal divider. *A*, right bronchus; *B*, left bronchus; *C*, main balloon; *D*, left bronchial balloon; *E*, right bronchus lumen; *F*, left bronchus lumen

breathing than other tubes, thus appearing particularly suitable for spontaneously breathing patients (see circuits for differential continuous positive airway pressure, CPAP).

Selective Bronchial Intubation

Whatever the model of the tube, the largest size compatible with the diameter of the airway should always be used. In our experience, the 39Ch and 37Ch are most often suitable for male and female patients, respectively. Some use topical anesthesia of the upper airways, glottis, and trachea in a lightly sedated patient for selective bronchial intubation.

An alternative technique is based upon neuroleptoanalgesia, short-acting barbiturates, and a depolarizing muscle relaxant. Both techniques have advantages and drawbacks.

In our opinion, the combination of anesthesia and muscle paralysis allows a more rapid intubation and limits the risk of autonomic reflexes, always dangerous in a critically ill patient. Once the glottis had been visualized, the biluminal tube is orotracheally inserted by progressing along the airway until the sensation of an obstacle is felt: the tracheal and bronchial cuffs are then inflated.

The correct position of the tube can be assessed in a number of ways, including:

1. Auscultation of the two lungs during simultaneous inflation.
2. Alternate clamping of the tracheal and bronchial lumen.
3. Alternative connection of one lumen to a water trap or to a small rubber bag while ventilating the other, the appearance of air bubbles or the inflation of the bag both revealing an insufficient bronchial seal.
4. Selective fibrobronchoscopy through the tracheal lumen.

In case of incorrect position the tube should be pulled back a few centimeters after deflation of the cuffs, and then reinserted. The correct position of the left bronchial lumen should always be confirmed by a chest radiography. Before fixation, the position of the tube at the mouth should be clearly marked, thus permitting rapid detection of any accidental displacement and easier positioning on reinsertion.

Assessment of the Functional Gradient

The functional separation of the two lungs with a good endobronchial seal achieves an important goal which allows the assessment of the functional gradient existing between the injured and the healthy parenchyma. This permits a number of bedside determinations: differential tidal volume (V_t) distribution, differential pressure/volume (P/V) loops (Fig. 3), selective airways resistance, and differential capnography. Further information can be obtained with more sophisticated techniques employing radioactive tracers or the computing of inert gases retention/excretion ratios: the latter, however, can not be employed routinely as it is both difficult to perform and time-consuming.

Whatever the technique employed, once the entity of the functional gradient has been assessed, the two lungs can be treated with the most appropriate combination of ventilatory supports. As a general rule, the healthy lung should be managed in such a way so to avoid as much iatrogenic damage as possible. In Fig. 7.3, for example, differential PEEP should be employed, starting with 12 cm H_2O for the right lung and a "prophylactic" PEEP of 4–5 cm H_2O in the left lung.

In general, after assessment of the functional gradient, selection of the combination of techniques of ventilatory support will fall into three main categories:

1. Patients with unilateral ALI and alveolar hypoventilation: in these subjects the selected ILV mode should provide a double CPPV circuit with differential PEEP values.
2. Patients with unilateral ALI and normo- or hypocapnea: these patients do not need to be ventilated, but will often improve if an adequate continuous

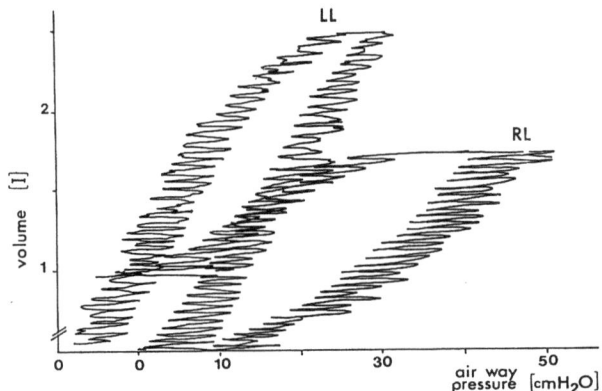

Fig. 3. Single lung pressure-volume traces (synringe technique). *LL* left lung; *RL* right lung

distending pressure is applied to the diseased lung, suggesting a circuit for differential CPAP.

3. Patients with unilateral ALI complicated by a bronchopleural fistula: in these cases it is often necessary to employ unilateral high frequency jet ventilation to manage this clinical problem.

In the next section a number of different circuits for ILV will be described as well as the modalities for their use.

Circuits for ILV

It is possible to divide the various circuits for ILV into three main categories:

1. Circuits with a single ventilator.
2. Circuits with two ventilators.
3. Circuits for spontaneous ventilation.

Circuits with a Single Ventilator

In this group, differential ventilation is provided by a special circuit inserted between the ventilator and the patient. Powner et al. (1977) have described a prototype, and subsequently Cavanilles et al. (1979) developed it as illustrated in Fig. 4. A selective inspiratory resistance allows tidal volume to be distributed to each lung according to the resistance and compliance of the parenchyma. It is possible to vary the PEEP level separately, as each lung has its expiratory limb. This circuit is not difficult to assemble, its main advantage being the use of a single ventilator. In complex situations, however, with its modulation potential limited

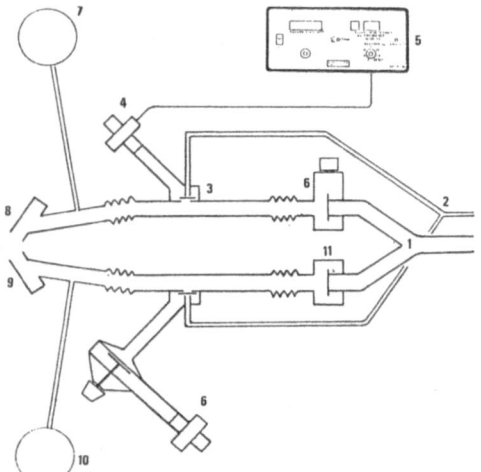

Fig. 4. Selective ventilation distribution circuit. *1*, Y piece; *2*, division of the expiratory valves line; *3*, expiratory (mushroom) valves; *4* and *6*, expiratory spirometers; *5*, capnography; *7* and *10*, pressure port; *8* and *9*, adapters to the Carlens tube

to VT and PEEP, it may not be sufficient to manage the pathological condition. More recently, Yamamura et al. (1985) have proposed some modifications to improve performance. Further clinical applications and experiences are needed before a definite statement can be made about the efficacy of this new circuit.

Circuits with Two Ventilators

The circuits for ILV that employ the coupling of two ventilators allow a broader spectrum of modulation of ventilatory parameters, as well as increased monitoring possibilities. The first authors to introduce these circuits into clinical use were greatly concerned about the synchronization of the two ventilators (Carlon et al. 1978b; Ray et al. 1978). The provision of respiratory cycles of the same duration, although with different Vt, I/E, and PEEP was thought superior in terms of hemodynamic tolerance. More recently, however, Hillman and Barber (1980) have demonstrated that asynchronous independent lung ventilation (ALIV) was able to maintain stable hemodynamic function while allowing for greater flexibility. The controversy about the value of synchronization seems more related to differing local facilities than to a real hemodynamic problem, at least in adults (Crimi et al. 1985; Marraro et al. 1986). However, electronic synchronization via a special cable (servo 900C "master and slave," Siemens Elema) seems not only reassuring from the clinical standpoint but also open new possibilities for further investigation of the pathophysiology of nonhomogeneous lung pathology. The nonsynchronization of the two ventilators is of course mandatory in ILV circuits providing unilateral HFPPV (Miranda et al. 1981) of HFJV (Crimi et al. 1986); with both techniques, hemodynamic good tolerance has been reported (Miranda et al. 1981; Crimi et al. 1986).

Circuits for Spontaneous Ventilation

Originally introduced by Venus et al. (1980), these circuits providing differential CPAP have not had as broad an application as they might due to unresolved management problems. The main concerns have been achieving appropriate sedation to combine adequate alveolar ventilation with obtundation of the pharyngeal reflexes and to overcome the increase of the resistive load to ventilation induced by the relatively narrow tubes. This notwithstanding, good results have been reported with this technique (Crimi et al. 1986), which appears easy to use. In this context, the previously mentioned possibility of employing a double lumen tracheostomy tube may contribute to the increased usage of this interesting ILV technique.

Monitoring ILV

This is a very important part of ILV management as proper monitoring allows rapid detection of modifications in alveolar gas exchange and tailoring of the ventilatory parameters to the functional conditions of the lung parenchyma.

Monitoring of ILV includes standard determinations (blood gas analysis, chest radiographs, airway pressures, selective expired VT), measurements of the mechanical properties of the lungs (selective P/V loops), and on-line evaluation of selective CO_2 washout. A pulmonary artery catheter is mandatory for the assessment of the hemodynamic function. The information gathered from these monitoring procedures is the key to safe management of ILV.

As an example, unilateral increase of peak airway pressure accompanying an altered capnogram rapidly diagnoses an acute obstruction of the ipsilateral lumen; on the other hand, the evidence of selective compliance values steadily improving is one of the best indices of the efficacy of treatment. In our experience, static compliance values differing by less than 30% are a good indication for the discontinuation of ILV.

Complications

Although very efficient, ILV is not an easy technique to manage. Close observation and skillful nursing are required for a successful outcome. Complications are best prevented, but when they do occur they must be treated rapidly. Obstruction of either lumen by tracheobronchial secretions should be prevented by careful humidification of the gas mixture and by frequent suctioning with catheters of appropriate shape and rigidity. The dislocation of the biluminal tubes is a particularly dangerous complication leading to alveolar hypoventilation and possible total airway obstruction by the bronchial cuff. Apart from the case of inadequate fixation, this complication may be precipitated by the enhanced pharyngeal reflexes of oral intubation. For this reason, patients should be moderately sedated, although the degree may be determined by the amount of spontaneous breathing that is permissible. If not, muscle paralysis may be preferable.

In our experience, fiberoptic bronchoscopy at extubation has never revealed signs of macroscopic damage to the tracheobronchial mucosa, even after long periods of ILV.

Results

As stated in the beginning, a rigorous evaluation of the results obtained with ILV is not possible, due to the relative scarcity of cases, the absence of comparative, randomized studies, and the great variability of the techniques employed. In the most favorable cases, the duration of ILV appears to be very short, as evidenced by its effectiveness when correctly indicated and managed. In most instances ILV can be demonstrated to manage patients with ALI effectively, irrespective of the final outcome; in the reported serie of cases, death was secondary to extrapulmonary causes.

In patients with unilateral lung lesion associated with bronchopleural fistula, ILV high frequency jet ventilation (HFJV) may be the treatment of choice. Rapid closure of the fistula is not always achieved, under conventional methods of ventilation, owing to the differing needs for parenchymal inflation in ALI versus the demand for a decrease in alveolar pressure to prevent air leak. In our experience, however, unilateral HFJV has led to a significant diminution of the air leak immediately with subsequent healing after a few hours.

When ILV is indicated for hemodynamic disturbances, satisfactory cardiovascular function can be restored immediately after the initiation of the differential ventilation, either with synchronous or asynchronous ventilators. This beneficial effect of ILV on the hemodynamics is of particular importance, as the final outcome of many patients with unilateral ALI often depends upon the duration of cardiovascular failure induced by conventional ventilatory support.

No major side effects of ILV have been reported from the authors listed in Table 1, even during the longest periods of treatment.

Conclusions

Although burdened by various problems of equipment and management, ILV represents the only solution to unilateral ALI refractory to both conventional ventilation and the lateral decubitus position. When properly used, ILV may resolve the injury rapidly with resulting correction of the interpulmonary functional gradient and a spectacular improvement in the patient's clinical condition. Future improvement in materials will surely lead to safer clinical management with this technique and to broader application.

References

Baehrendtz S, Hedenstierna G (1984) Differential ventilation and selective positive end expiratory pressure: effects on patients with acute bilateral lung disease. Anesthesiology 61:511–517

Benumof JL (1978) Mechanism of decreased blood flow to atelectasic lung. J Appl Physiol 46:1047

Carlon GG, Kahn R, Howland W, Baron R, Ramaker J (1978a) Acute life threatening ventilation-perfusion inequality: an indication for independent lung ventilation. Crit Care Med 6:380–383

Carlon GC, Ray C, Klein R (1978b) Criteria for selective PEEP and independent synchronized ventilation of each lung. Chest 74:501

Cavanilles JM, Garrigosa F, Oncins JR (1979) A selective ventilation distribution circuit. Intensive Care Med 5:95–98

Crimi G, Conti, G, Mattia C, Gasparetto A (1985) The management of unilateral acute lung injury. Anaesthesiol Intensivmed 178:112–115

Crimi G, Candiani A, Conti G, Mattia C, Gasparetto A (1986) Clinical applications of independent lung ventilation with unilateral high frequency jet ventilation. Intensive Care Med 12:90–94

Crimi G, Conti G, Bufi M, Antonelli M, Mattia C, Gasparetto A (1987) Clinical application of differential CPAP in the treatment of unilateral acute lung injury. Intensive Care Med 13:416–418

Fishman AP (1976) Hypoxia on the pulmonary circulation: how and where it acts. Circ Res 38:221

Hedenstierna G, Baehrendtz S, Klingstedt C, et al. (1984) Ventilation and perfusion of each lung during differential ventilation with selective PEEP. Anesthesiology 61:369–376

Hillman K, Barber JD (1980) Asynchronous independent lung ventilation. Crit Care Med 8:390–395

Marraro G, Marinari M, Rataggi M, Colnaghi E (1986) Synchronized independent lung ventilation (Silv) and selective PEEP: effects on children with lung pathology with monolateral prevalence. Intensive Care Med 12:273

Miranda DR, Stoutenbeek C, Kingma L (1981) Differential lung ventilation with HFPPV. Intensive Care Med 7:139–141

Powner DJ, Gross B, Grenvik A (1977) Differential lung ventilation with PEEP in the treatment of unilateral pneumonia. Crit Care Med 5:170–172

Ray C, Carlon CG, Miodownik S, Goldiner PL (1978) A method of synchronizing two MA1 ventilators for independent lung ventilation (Abstr). Crit Care Med 6:99

Venus B, Pratap KS, Op'Tholt T (1980) Treatment of unilateral pulmonary insufficiency by selective administration of continuous positive airway pressure through a double lumen tube. Anesthesiology 52:74–77

Yamamura T, Furukuda H, Saito Y (1985) A single-unit device for differential lung ventilation with only one anesthesia machine. Anesth Analg 64:1017–26

Ventilation in Severe ARDS:
Inverted Ratio Ventilation and CO_2 Removal[1]

L. Gattinoni, D. Mascheroni, M. Borelli, E. Basilico, and A. Pesenti

The incidence of adult acute respiratory distress syndrome (ARDS) in Western Europe is unknown. However, inferring from data available in the USA (Petty and Newmann 1978) and considering the population of the USA and Western Europe to be equivalent as a first approximation, the number of ARDS cases should be close to 150 000. The mortality rate, in different reported series ranges from 15% (Gallagher et al. 1978) to 90% (Zapol et al. 1979), according to the patient population in the study.

There is general agreement that the average mortality rate is about 50% (Hudson 1982) which indicates that the therapy of what is called ARDS is still an unsolved problem. Indeed, there has been a continuous search for new therapeutic approaches. In the past few years, two main research directions in ARDS have evolved, the first aimed at identifying the biological determinants of the lesions occurring in this syndrome (Petty and Fowler 1982; Rinaldo and Rogers 1982) and the second aimed at the improvement of clinical outcome through modifications of the respiratory assistance (Shapiro et al. 1983). The identification of biological intermediates of the basic lesion of ARDS should allow, in the future, determination of the appropriate pharmacological means to prevent or to stop the disease course, i.e., to really cure the ARDS. It is more difficult to define exactly what may be expected in the form of possible "improvement" in respiratory support. It is reasonable to state that the main goal of respiratory treatment is to "buy" enough time for possible lung healing, by providing viable gas exchange and preventing further damage to the pulmonary structures.

The ideal respiratory support should be one where the hypothetical iatrogenic damage/gas exchange ratio is kept as low as possible. We will discuss whether this risk/benefit ratio may be improved by newer forms of respiratory support, i.e., inverted ratio ventilation (IRV) and extracorporeal CO_2 removal ($ECCO_2R$).

[1] This work has been in part support by C.N.R. grant no. 84.02098.57, Rome, December 1984

Current Respiratory Treatment of ARDS

It is worth emphasizing that all respiratory assistance is symptomatic treatment, where the common end point is to assure adequate gas exchange, which is not necessarily related to either lung healing or to the final outcome. There is general agreement that survival from ARDS is related mainly to resolution of the underlying disease, and strictly linked to the number of failing organs other than the lungs (National Heart and Lung Institute 1974). If the basic disease (e.g., sepsis, pancreatitis) cannot be corrected by natural evolution, pharmacology, or surgery, the prognosis is poor, irrespective of the effectiveness of respiratory assistance. However, it is possible that the current respiratory treatment of ARDS, i.e., continuous positive pressure ventilation (CPPV) used worldwide as the main form of respiratory assistance, may be a factor which per se adds to lung pathology, thus, contributing an additional increase in mortality. The 'natural history" of ARDS should, more correctly, be called the "natural history of ARDS + CPPV" where the effects of CPPV are still the undermined factor. High FiO_2, high pressures, and high ventilation are the main characteristics of mechanical ventilation (MV) in ARDS. Let us first briefly consider the effects of each of these factors on normal, healthy lungs.

Mechanical Ventilation and Healthy Lungs

MV in healthy lungs is a safe technique. The day by day experience in the operating room with short-term anesthesia and prolonged MV in patients with neuromuscular disease clearly show that the "normal" MV of the "normal lung" is usually performed without side effects of clinical relevance.

However, in these conditions the ventilated lungs are normal, with normal volumes and compliance, and gas exchange is also in the normal range. Indeed FiO_2 is not usually higher than 0.30–0.40. The peak pressure is rather low (usually below 20 cm H_2O), and the amount of ventilation required to clear the CO_2 production is still in the normal range (6–8 l/min^{-1}). The Tidal volume (VT)/functional residual capacity (FRC) ratio (1:4, 1:5) is normal and the "specific" ventilation, i.e., the amount of ventilation per unit of lung volume is kept within the physiological range. However, if FiO_2 is elevated, peak pressure increased, or specific ventilation higher than the normal, the safety of MV in the normal lung may be questionable.

Inspired Oxygen Fraction

Oxygen toxicity to the lungs was first described by Smith in 1899 and is widely recognized. In 1965, Linton et al. described, in patients with previously normal lungs and neuromuscular disease, "respirator lung" where clinical and pathological changes were similar to those observed in ARDS patients. Unfortunately, the FiO_2 in use was not reported. However, 2 years later, after studying 70 patients on MV, Nash et al. (1967) concluded that an inspired oxygen concentration higher than 90% was the only parameter correlated with pathological changes characteristics of ARDS.

It is not appropriate to discuss here oxygen toxicity or its possible relationship with humidification. For our purposes, it is sufficient to note that animal studies clearly show the potential danger of oxygen in the healthy lung (Deneke and Fanburg 1982). However, what may be considered absolutely "safe" oxygen concentration in the critically ill has yet to be determined.

High Peak Pressure in Healthy Lungs

There is consistent evidence that high peak pressure in healthy lungs may also create a pulmonary damage such as edema and increased alveolar surface tension with increased and peripheral airway collapse. These effects, different from oxygen toxicity, are seldom recognized. Greenfield et al. (1964) showed progressive lung damage in healthy dogs subjected to peak pressures of 26–32 cm H_2O; after 1.5–3.5 h of MV on room air, there was evidence of pulmonary edema. After 24 h, they found alterations in lung surfactant. Vascular injury, atelectasis, hyaline membranes, and decreased lung surfactant were found by Barsch et al. (1970) after 22–70 of MV with peak pressures of 20–34 cmH_2O, FiO_2 being 0.21 or 1.0. Fariday et al. (1966) in isolated healthy goat lungs found decreased compliance and high surface tension, directly correlated with size and duration of MV. Wyszgrodski et al. (1975) had the same results in intact cats. Pulmonary damage, edema, and decreased compliance were found by Webb and Tierney (1974) in rats after 1 h of MV with a peak pressure of 45 cm H_2O. Kolobow et al. (unpublished studies) in 1983 and 1984, in a large series of healthy sleep, used 48 h of MV with a FiO_2 of 0.4 and peak pressure of 30 cm H_2O to induce parenchymal respiratory failure. Diffuse X-ray alterations, derangements in pulmonary mechanics, and impairment in gas exchange were the consistent findings of these studies.

Summarizing, it appears likely that MV, when delivered at high peak pressure (though 30 cm H_2O in the ICU setting is considered "safe") may cause damage to the lung. It is still unclear if the peak pressure is the only factor responsible for these alterations. The possible role of positive end-expiratory pressure (PEEP) or mean airway pressure (MPAW) has yet to be determined.

Hyperventilation in the Healthy Lung

Faridy et al. (1966) showed that ventilation of excised lungs at 30%–50% of maximum lung volume caused a decrease in compliance within 3 h, while lungs ventilated at 10% of maximum lung volume maintained normal elasticity. We and McClenahan and Urthowstri (1967) have both reported that the increase in elastic recoil was proportional to the VT and to the respiratory rate.

Webb and Tierney (1974) using large tidel volume (though with bush peak pressure) found in rat lungs perimicrovascular and alveolar edema. Similar observations were reported by Thet and Alvarez (1982). Mascheroni et al. (1985)

in an attempt to separate the effects of hyperventilation per se and high peak pressures (normally employed to obtain hyperventilation), injected sodium salicylate into the cisterna magna of healthy sheep. This caused spontaneous ventilation, without systemic acidosis, resulting over the following 12 h in progressive fall of PaO_2, lung commpliance, and an increase in alveolar-arterial PO_2 gradient. At autopsy, the lungs were severely atelectatic (over 30% of the area). In the control animals, hyperventilation was prevented by use of paralysis and "normal-volume-pressure" MV. Gas exchange remained within normal limits and no alterations were found at autopsy.

Dreyfuss et al. (1985) have shown that MV with large tidal volume results in lung damage (permeability type edema) whether obtained with high peak (45 cm H_2O), positive pressure MV, or negative external pressure ("iron lung"). However, during high peak positive pressure MV, the lung damage was prevented when avoiding large tidal volume excursion by chest-abdominal strapping (Dreyfuss et al. 1986). All these findings suggest that hyperventilation is in itself a mechanism of lung damage; however, very little is known about the mechanisms involved.

Kolobow et al. (1981) showed that local alkalosis caused severe lung damage within 2–8 h. The alkalosis was induced in healthy sheep by ventilating them while on total venoarterial bypass. The $\dot{V}A/\dot{Q}$ of the lung was thus extremely elevated with an increase in local pH. The damage was prevented, in the same model, by adding 3% CO_2 into the ventilating gas mixture.

Alterations in surfactant may also be a mechanism of hyperventilation-induced lung damage. Faridy et al. (1966) suggested that surfactant alterations could be caused by repeated overcompression of the layer which occurs during hyperventilation. In this situation, increased surfactant clearance through the airways was also observed (Faridy 1971). Moderate hyperventilation was able to damage lungs in which subclinical alterations of surfactant were induced by starvation (Thet and Alvarez 1982). Finally, the overdistention of lung cells and structures may also be considered as possible injurious factors.

In conclusion, it may well be possible that hyperventilation injures the healthy lung. It should, however, be noted that the amount of ventilation which produced lung damage in these reported studies (two to three times normal) is likely to be used in ARDS patients.

Summarizing, the factors leading to potential damage to lung structures— FiO_2 peak pressure, and hyperventilation are all components of current respiratory treatment of ARDS. We will describe, in more detail, what may be the impact of CPPV in ARDS lungs.

Lung Physiology in ARDS

In full-blown ARDS, the lung is not homogeneously diseased. Different pathological lesions, e.g., fibrosis of different degrees, interstitial/alveolar edema, vascular thrombosis and hyaline membranes, may coexist in the same lung with normally structured areas. Plain chest films or, better, computed tomography

(CT) scanning, may show the presence of "healthy" areas in close proximity to "high density" parenchymal structures. We may indeed hypothesize, from a functional and simplified point of view, that the ARDS lung is basically a composite mixture of three different "areas": (a) diseased, (b) recruitable, and (c) healthy.

Diseased Areas. These are areas of alveolar and/or vascular occlusion, where ventilation and/or perfusion are completely absent. The functional equivalent would be the right to left shunt and the alveolar dead space. The existence of such areas is well documented by biopsy or autopsy pulmonary specimens. No amount of positive pressure would make these areas available for gas exchange until the basic lesions are naturally solved.

Recruitable Areas. These may be considered as the "potentially workable" areas, where respiratory assistance may produce the most dramatic effects. However, the presence of such areas is not consistent and they tend to disappear in the late stages of ARDS (Matamis et al. 1984). The possibility of recruitment may be inferred by radiology and CT scanning, showing the appearance of newly aerated areas when increasing PEEP. More generally, the effectiveness of PEEP is mainly attributed to "recruitment," and the presence of a clear inflection point on the P-V curve of the lung is further support for this view (Lemaire et al. 1980). Once sufficient positive pressure is applied and the peripheral airways kept open, gas exchange may take place in the recruited area, and both oxygenation and CO_2 clearance are improved.

Healthy Areas. Pathological samples, radiology, and CT scanning may document morphologically the presence of areas in an ARDS lung unaffected by the disease process. Functionally, the specific compliance of the ARDS lung (i.e., lung compliance/FRC) has been found within the normal range in ARDS patients (Suter et al. 1978; Gattinoni et al. 1982), meaning that the mechanical characteristics of the residual healthy areas probably remain normal.

Though this is a simplified model, the basic assumptions appear reasonable and fit with the available pathological and functional data.

Gas Exchange in ARDS

Gas exchange in ARDS takes place only in recruited and healthy areas, which may be, in severe ARDS, as low as 20%–30% of normal lung volume. The entire respiratory burden must therefore be accomplished in this reduced volume with consequently reduced compliance. To maintain oxygenation, elevated FiO_2, MPAW, and PEEP are required. To maintain a normal $PaCO_2$, the specific ventilation is greatly increased (VT/FRC ratio up to ten times the normal) with consequently elevated peak pressures. All these factors have been shown, as previously discussed, to cause damage in the remaining healthy lung. Moreover, almost all organ systems may be impaired by high-pressure volume ventilation, which is also responsible for the spectrum of barotrauma lesions.

Search for "Optimal" Respiratory Assistance in ARDS

It is evident, from the above considerations, that MV in ARDS is always a compromise between the need to prolong life by maintaining a viable gas exchange and the iatrogenic damage induced by the treatment on the residual healthy areas of the pulmonary parenchyma. The search for "optimal" respiratory therapy should always consider a hypothetical risk/benefic ratio where the benefit is the gas exchange (the goal of the treatment) and the cost is possible iatrogenic damage.

Both halves of the ratio (with risk including: FiO_2, peak pressure, hyperventilation, PEEP (?), and MPAW (?) and Benefit being: effective gas exchange) must be considered when introducing alternative forms of respiratory assistance. What is the relationship between the risk and benefit, and what is currently available to improve this ratio?

To improve oxygenation, there are several available techniques:

1. *Increase FiO_2.* Conventionally, the upper limit of safety for FiO_2 is 0.6, 0.4 being considered absolutely safe, provided there is optimal gas humidification.
2. *Increase airway pressure.* As discussed, the main function of positive pressure is to recruit new areas for gas exchange and to keep them open. Once a "minimal PEEP" is provided (Lemaire et al. 1981), oxygenation is mainly a function of MPAW (Pesenti et al. 1990) though the role of peak pressure may be of some importance (Suter et al. 1978), however, the same mean airway pressure may be delivered with a different combination of I:E ratio and PEEP. Increasing the I:E ratio allows a decrease in the peak pressure, while maintaining constant MPAW. For a given MPAW, the higher the I:E ratio, the lower the peak pressure and PEEP, and the risk/benefit ratio may decrease.
3. *Improved $\dot{V}a/\dot{Q}$ distribution.* For a given set of FiO_2 and MPAW, oxygenation may be further improved only through modification of regional $\dot{V}a/\dot{Q}s$. For a given cardiac output, better gas distribution should result in better gas exchange. While in severe ARDS the importance of $\dot{V}a/\dot{Q}$ maldistribution is questionable (Dantzker et al. 1979), the hypoxemia being almost entirely due to a true shunt, in less severe ARDS the maldistribution component appears to be of clinical relevance (Pesenti et al. 1983).

With the exception of FiO_2, all the factors involved in oxygenation also play a role in the CO_2 clearance, including:

1. *Pressures.* Total ventilation recruitment of new areas for gas exchange also improves CO_2 clearance. Retention, which is sometimes observed when increasing PEEP or MPAW, is probably related to overinflation of previously open areas (no recruitment), suggesting an excessive pressure load (Tuler 1983). CO_2 exchange, in this view, has been proposed as a "tool" to tailor the PEEP level (Murray et al. 1984).
2. *$\dot{V}a/\dot{Q}$ distribution.* A real improvement of the regional $\dot{V}a/\dot{Q}$ ratio improves the CO_2 clearance, for the same reasons.

3. *Ventilation.* The most important determinant of CO_2 clearance, however, remains the adequacy of ventilation. The increase in specific ventilation (i.e., local hyperventilation) is the unavoidable cost to be paid in ARDS to maintain $PaCO_2$ with in a normal range.

Summarizing, for a given set of "iatrogenic risks" or "costs," the risk/benefit ratio may be improved only by modification of gas distribution through the lung. Alternatively, for a given gas exchange, the ratio may be improved if peak pressures are decreased or hyperventilation abolished. The rationale for IRV and $ECCO_2R$, as will be discussed in detail, is to improve both the terms of the risk/benefit ratio by (a) improving gas distribution, (b) decreasing the peak pressure, and (c) completely abolishing the need for ventilation in the case of $ECCO_2R$.

Inverted Ratio Ventilation (see chapter by J. B. Andersen)

The I/E ratio is defined as the quotient between the inspiration time (including the inspiratory hold) and expiration time (including the expiratory pause). During MV, the I/E is generally set at 1:2 (Safar 1965). The inversion of the I/E ratio (IRV) was first clinically proposed by Reynolds (1971) for the respiratory treatment of infant hyaline membrane disease. Some years later, Baum et al. (1980) and Lachmann et al. (1980) applied IRV in the treatment of ARDS. Baum et al. (1980) used volume controlled IRV 4:1 (independent variables being the inspiratory square wave flow, VT, and respiratory rate). The resultant peak pressure and MPAW were therefore dependent on the patient's lung compliance. In contrast, Lachmann et al. (1980) applied pressure controlled IRV 4:1 (independent variables being pressure limit and "decelerated" inspiratory flow with inspiratory hold). Thus, the minute ventilation, for a given peak pressure limit, was dependent on the patient's lung compliance.

Both Baum et al. (1980) and Lachmann et al. (1980), as well as Reynolds (1971) in infants, found a consistent improvement in oxygenation, a decrease in Vd/Vt, a reduced barotrauma, and a reduced hemodynamic impairment. These findings were confirmed in successive clinical reports (Gattinoni et al. 1984; Osswald et al. 1981).

The reported clinical advantages of IRV may be summarized as follows:

1. *Increase in CO_2 clearance.* This has been reported by most authors both in experimental and clinical settings (Cheney Burnam 1971; Fulheihan et al. 1976; Knelson et al. 1970). The reduction of Vd/Vt during IRV has been recognized for a long time and appears to be unequivocal (Sykes and Lumley 1969). The decrease in Vd/Vt may allow a reduction in minute ventilation with a consequent decrease in peak pressure and MPAW.
2. Improved oxygenation. Most authors have found an improvement in oxygenation with IRV. However, the underlying mechanism(s) is (are) still unclear and an increase in MPAW is likely to play an important role (this topic will be discussed later).

Therefore, the potential of IRV is to maintain effective gas exchange while reducing peak pressure and/or PEEP (at constant MPAW and ventilation) or to reduce even MPAW and ventilation, due to a decrease in Vd/Vt. All these mechanisms decrease the iatrogenic risk of ventilation by decreasing barotrauma. The histological data of Lachmann, in an experimental setting of a lung lavage model of ARDS, support this hypothesis (Knelson et al. 1970).

The question is whether IRV can actually improve the gas exchange at a lower iatrogenic cost. Unfortunately, IRV is generally compared with CPPV at the same PEEP level, and the values of MPAW are not usually reported. However, the increase in I/E ratio impressively increases the MPAW (Pesenti et al. 1990). In a recent study (Gattinoni et al. 1990), we compared CPPV and IRV at the same MPAW and equal minute ventilation: gas exchange and hemodynamics were identical. PEEP and peak pressure were lower in the IRV setting, and this may indeed be an advantage during the long term. Cole et al. (1984) recently reported great advantages of IRV, compared with CPPV and a lower MPAW, with the I/E being not 4:1, but 1.7:1. In this case, the cost/benefit ratio should really decrease and IRV should be a valid alternative to conventional ventilation for a given MPAW.

The IRV may improve oxygenation and CO_2 removal through mechanisms other than increase in airway pressure, including:

1. *Improvement of gas distribution.* Such a mechanism is suggested to play a role especially in the presence of "slow alveoli", with increased time constant (TC, compliance × resistance) (Mute et al. 1983). In the areas with increased resistance (increased TC), ventilation should improve with prolonged inspiration time. On the other hand, if compliance is decreased, TC is decreased and IRV would not improve gas distribution. Moreover, the overall ventilation may improve in areas at elevated TC only with an absolute increase in inspiratory time (dependent not only on the I/E ratio, but also on the product of the I/E ratio and respiratory rate).
2. "Auto-PEEP." If expiration time is decreased to a certain limit, "auto-PEEP" (Pepe and Martin 1982) (i.e., gas trapping) may be generated, since not enough time is left for complete deflation of the lungs. The term "individual PEEP" has been used to describe the gas trapping occurring in areas with expiratory TC higher than normal. In these areas, higher PEEP is "regionally" maintained while the areas with lower TC completely deflate to the selected PEEP (i.e., individual PEEP is higher than selected PEEP). Once again, only areas with relatively normal or high compliance and increased resistance may present gas trapping.

In the areas with low compliance auto-PEEP is unlikely to occur. Indeed, no report in the literature has correlated "auto-PEEP" or "individual-PEEP" with an improvement in gas exchange. Moreover, this phenomenon is potentially dangerous (lung ruptures) and explains the general concern of many authors in using an elevated I/E ratio.

Nevertheless, IRV presents some potential advantages compared with CPPV: lower peak and PEEP at the same MPAW, the possibility of decreasing minute ventilation, and possible improvement in gas distribution. All these factors decrease the cost/benefit of mechanical ventilation.

Unfortunately, the danger of gas trapping may overcome the potential advantages in particular patients (Conors et al. 1981). It is our opinion that the "classical" IRV (4:1) should be avoided, except, maybe, as a temporary tool to improve oxygenation (Gattinoni et al. 1984). IRV with a ratio from 1:1 to 3:1 is more likely to reduce barotrauma, compared with CPPV at similar MPAW. The effectiveness of this technique must be evaluated in each patient, with a short trial and careful monitoring of gas exchange, pulmonary mechanics, and hemodynamics.

Extracorporeal CO_2 Removal

Extracorporal CO_2 removal is a technique of respiratory assistance based on the "lung rest" concept (Gattinoni et al. 1983a): the diseased lungs are kept motionless, and ventilated two to three times per minute at limited peak pressure. Oxygenation is accomplished through "apneic oxygenation" (Frumin et al. 1959) and CO_2 is removed extracorporeally through an artificial lung by a venovenous bypass.

This technique was introduced clinically in 1980 (Gattinani et al. 1980a) after extensive experimental work. Animal studies have shown the following:

1. Extracorporeal CO_2 removal in healthy awake animals controls pulmonary ventilation, which is decreased proportionally to the percent of minute CO_2 production removed by artificial means. The FiO_2 must be raised to compensate for the resultant hypoventilation (Kolobow et al. 1977). The same finding is commonly observed in dialysed patients (Martin 1980), where some CO_2 is cleared through the artificial kidneys. Control of breathing was also studied in animals mechanically ventilated: the decrease in mechanical ventilation required to maintain a constant $PaCO_2$ was proportional to the increase in extracorporeal CO_2 removal (Gattinoni et al. 1978a).
2. It is possible to maintain normal oxygenation and $PaCO_2$ in apneic animals when the total minute CO_2 production is cleared through the artificial lungs and an amount of oxygen equal to oxygen consumption is directly supplied into the trachea (Kolobow et al. 1978). However, the levels of oxygenation, in this setting, are MPAW dependent, as low MPAW (5 cm H_2O) results, after 24 h, in a decreased FRC. FRC may be restored after manual ventilation for a short time. If the MPAW is higher (up to 20 cm H_2O), no decrease in oxygenation is observed (Gattinoni et al. 1979). The FRC drop may also be prevented if, in the apnea model, "sighs" (two to three per minute) are superimposed. This is what is called low frequency positive pressure ventilation with extracorporeal CO_2 removal (LFPPV-$ECCO_2R$) (Gattinoni et al. 1978b). LFPPV-$ECCO_2R$ has shown better hemodynamics and renal func-

tion compared with CPPV (Gattinoni et al. 1980b), and was chosen instead of apnea as the form of respiratory assistance for clinical application.

LFPPV-ECCO$_2$R Technique

This technique has been described in detail elsewhere (Pesenti et al. 1981), and will only be summarized here.

Extracorporeal Circuit

The drainage catheter is positioned in the inferior vena cava (7–8 cm below the diaphragm). The vascular access, dependent on the vein size, is through the long saphenous (single lumen catheter) or through the common femoral vein (double lumen catheter) (Pesenti et al. 1982). Blood returns to the inferior vena cava 2 cm below the diaphragm through the inner catheter of the double lumen catheter or through the saphenous vein catheter inserted in the other side. The saphenosaphenous cannulation, when feasible, is simpler than femoral cannulation, and provides adequate flow (1.5–2.5 $1 \cdot min^{-1}$). The blood is collected by gravity into a collapsable reservoir and with a roller pump pumped through two artificial lungs, suitable for long-term use (SCI Med-Kolobow), connected in series, and returned to the patient.

The artificial lungs are ventilated with an air/oxygen mixture, according to clinical need. The entire extracorporeal circuit is enclosed in a thermostated compact console (Kontron LSS 6000). Essential monitoring is continuously displayed, and includes temperature, pressure across the artificial lungs, extracorporeal blood flow, and input blood oxygen saturation. Alarms and Servo control are provided for gas and blood flows, temperature, and pressures. The circuit is provided with suitable ports for hemodialysis and hemofiltration, if required (Gattinoni et al. 1983b).

Respiratory Circuit

The patient is connected to a ventilator which provides three to four cycles/min at limited pressure (25–45 cm H_2O). A small Teflon catheter is advanced, through a side port of the tracheal tube, directly into the carina and provides for oxygen consumption during the end expiratory pause. The level of positive pressure is set according to clinical needs.

Entry Criteria

The entry criteria are the following:

1. Gas exchange: PaO$_2$ lower than 50 mmHg with FiO$_2$: 1 and shunt fraction greater than 30% for 48 h when measured at PEEP 5 cm H_2O. These criteria,

used in the NIH ECMO study, correspond to a mortality greater than 90%
(National Heart and Lung Institute, 1979).
2. Total static lung compliance (TSLC) lower than $30\,ml/cm\ H_2O^{-1}$. The full
   discussion of these entry criteria is reported elsewhere (Gattinoni et al. 1984).

Clinical Procedure

The patient is paralyzed and under light anesthesia throughout the procedure.
Complete respiratory, hemodynamic, and coagulation monitoring is mandatory.
After the surgery, the patient is connected to the extracorporeal circuit and
$ECCO_2R$ begins. As the pulmonary ventilation is decreased to 3–4 breaths/min,
PEEP is raised to maintain MPAW at the same level as during the previous
CPPV period, to avoid sudden edema. FiO_2 is also maintained at the same
concentration. When consistent improvement in gas exchange is achieved
(usually after a few hours of LFPPV-$ECCO_2R$) the FiO_2 of the ventilator is
decreased and the artificial lungs are ventilated with room air. The pressures are
decreased when a PaO_2 greater than 100 mmHg is consistently recorded.
Weaning and decurarization start when the shunt fraction is lower than 20%, at
FiO_2 0.4, total lung capacity is greater than $30\,ml/cm\ H_2O$ (measured on inflation
limb of pressure volume curve, at 10 ml/kg volume), and chest X-ray shows a
consistent clearing. The patient is disconnected when effective gas exchange is
maintained in continuous positive airway pressure (CPAP) for 6–12 h without
extracorporeal gas exchange.

Clinical Results

Since 1980, more than 30 patients/year have been referred to our Institute from
other ICUS for extracorporeal support. Only 1/3 fulfilled the entry criteria and
underwent LFPPV-$ECCO_2R$. The patients have been retrospectively classified
as responders and nonresponders. Responders were those who showed consistent
improvement in lung function within 24–48 h from the beginning of LFPPV-

Table 1. Results of LFPPV-$ECCO_2R$

Pulmonary disease	Patients (n)	Responders	Nonresponders	Long-term survivors
Viral pneumonia	10	7 (70%)	3 (33%)	5 (50%)
Viral pneumonia in AIDS	2	0	2 (100%)	0
Bacterial pneumonia	8	7 (87.5%)	1 (12.5%)	5 (62.5%)
Toxic, septic, shock lung	5	4 (80%)	1 (20%)	4 (80%)
Pulmonary embolism	4	2 (50%)	2 (50%)	2 (50%)
Multiple trauma	9	5 (55.5%)	4 (44%)	2 (22.2%)
Total	38	25 (65.8%)	13 (34.2%)	18 (47.4%)

$ECCO_2R$. None of the patients survived who after 48 h of LFPPV-$ECCO_2R$ had not demonstrated signs of improvement. Confirmation by others is required; however, according to our data, the treatment should be stopped after 48–72 h if no response is recorded.

The clinical LFPPV-$ECCO_2R$ experience is largely limited to our Institute, though a few other patients have been treated in Berlin (Falke and colleagues), Marburg (Lennartz and colleagues), and Paris (F. Brunet and colleagues). To date, we have managed 38 ARDS patients. Among them 68% were responders and 18 are long-term survivors, with recovery of normal lung function in most cases. Table 1 shows the etiology, the response to the therapy, and the final outcome. The mean time on CPPV before connection to the bypass and the mean time of bypass are shown in Table 2. No significant differences were recorded in the duration of disease between responders and nonresponders. The mean time of LFPPV-$ECCO_2R$ for survivors was 5.31 ± 3.33 days. All but two patients had some degree of multiple systems organ failure when the bypass was initiated. Some patients survived with up to three organ failures other than the lung. No survivor was recorded with more than a total of four systems failures. Particularly, central nervous system failure had a bad prognosis. No differences in organ failure distribution between responders and nonresponders could be detected. The etiology did not discriminate between responders and nonresponders. However, a priori identification of the responder patients will be of great importance in defining the indications for this technique. The only difference we could find between responders and nonresponders before the connection was a significantly higher $PaCO_2$ (greater than 55 mmHg) in nonresponders compared with the responders (less than 50 mmHg), at comparable hemodynamic and total ventilation ($280 \, ml/kg^{-1} \, min^{-1}$).

It will be important to understand if this represents a different degree of the same pathological process or a different pathological process. The overall treatment during LFPPV-$ECCO_2R$ is basically the same for other critically ill patients. The only problem added is the necessity of continuous heparinization with the potential complications (Uziel et al. 1982). Staff requirements are increased: the nurse/patient ratio should be kept at 1:1; a doctor, familiar with the

Table 2. Duration of respiratory support

Pulmonary disease	Patients (n)	CPPV duration of prior to $ECCO_2R$ (days)	Duration of (days)
Viral pneumonia	10	4.15 ± 2.93	10.57 ± 8.53
Viral pneumonia in AIDS	2	-27 ± 22.63	7.79 ± 7.72
Bacterial pneumonia	8	14.29 ± 13.33	8.47 ± 7.17
Toxic, septic, shock lung	5	14.09 ± 23.82	3.58 ± 2.19
Pulmonary embolism	4	15.8 ± 22.81	5.58 ± 3.93
Multiple trauma	9	15 ± 12.76	8.98 ± 2.81
Total mean $\pm$ SD	38	15.06 ± 7.26	7.50 ± 2.52

extracorporeal apparatus is required to be on hand 24 h a day, and a surgeon and hematologist should be readily available. After more than 8000 h of LFPPV-$ECCO_2R$, we have not had a major technical accident which required removal of the bypass. LFPPV-$ECCO_2R$ appears to be a safe technique. One patient was on bypass for 31 days without complication. Cost analysis has shown that the mean daily cost of LEPPV-$ECCO_2R$ is double compared with that of routine management of a critically ill patient in ICU.

To date, we have not used LFPPV-$ECCO_2R$ as primary respiratory assistance, but only when CPAP, IMV, CPPV, IRV, and occasionally high frequency jet ventilation have failed to maintain effective gas exchange. There are several mechanisms by which the beneficial effect of LFPPV-$ECCO_2R$ may be explained. First, a significant amount of oxygen, approximatively 20%–30% of $\dot{V}O_2$, is provided by artificial lungs even when ventilated with room air. More interesting is the possible effect on gas exchange in the diseased lung: (a) apnea is the ideal form to provide even alveolar PO_2 distribution, and this has been demonstrated experimentally with LFPPV-$ECCO_2R$ (Green et al. 1983); (b) all the advantages of IRV, in terms of gas distribution may be translated to LFPPV-$ECCO_2R$ without the danger of gas trapping, as the time for deflation is longer. In terms of "iatrogenic cost" of LFPPV, the peak pressures are limited in amount and in number. FiO_2 may be decreased because of the artificial lungs, and the local hyperventilation is completely abolished. The cost/benefit or therapeutic ratio of respiratory assistance is greatly improved.

Finally, it may be that apnea, or simply withdrawal of CPPV, may influence fluid exchange in the diseased lung. Peters et al. (1988) and Knoch (1989), independently, have shown in human cases, a progressive decrease in extra-vascular lung water. The change in patient status within a few hours of LFPPV-$ECCO_2R$ is often dramatic. However, we do not know why some patients are nonresponders (34%). It is attractive to speculate that nonresponders are patients whose main pathology is in the microvascular system, in which case no form of ventilation may solve the problem.

Conclusion

If we accept the concept of considering the respiratory assistance in terms of cost/benefit, it is evident that both IRV and LFPPV-$ECCO_2R$ may very well not be only "last ditch" treatments but rather true alternative forms of respiratory support. All forms of ventilation may be considered in terms of risk/benefit ratio, since iatrogenic damage and the future of the lungs are equally as important as the gas exchange. However, compared with all other forms of respiratory assistance, where the entire respiratory burden must be assumed by the diseased lung, LFPPV-$ECCO_2R$ has the advantage, even in the most desperate situation, of giving an extra additional lung, thus, buying time and buffering the emergency. Moreover, the extra lung rests the diseased lung and may provide the opportunity to heal. Randomized studies are probably warranted to test this technique in less desperate situations, not as a "last resort," but as an alternative to current respiratory treatment.

References

Barsch J, Bibara C, Eggers GWN, Krumlofsky F, Sanit YW, Smith W, Smith Webster J (1970) Positive pressure as a cause of respirator induced lung disease. Ann Intern Med 72:810

Baum M, Benzer H, Mutz N, Pauser G, Tonczar L (1980) Inverted ratio ventilation (IRV). Die Rolle des Atemzeitverhältnisses in der Beatmung beim ARDS. Anaesthesist 29:592

Cheney F, Burnam C (1971) Effect of ventilatory pattern on oxygenation on pulmonary edema. J Appl Physiol 31:909

Cole AGH, Weller SF, Sykes MK (1984) Inverse ratio ventilation compared with PEEP in adult respiratory failure. Intensive Care Med 10:227

Conors A, McCaffree DR, Gray BA (1981) Effect of inspiratory flow rate on gas exchange during mechanical ventilation. Am Rev Respir Dis 124:537

Dantzker D, Brook CJ, Dehart P, Lynch JP, Weg JG (1979) Ventilation-perfusion distributions in adult respiratory distress syndrome. Am Rev Respir Dis 120:1039

Deneke SM, Fanburg BL (1988) Oxygen toxicity of the lung: an update. Br J Anaesth 54:737

Dreyfuss D, Basset G, Soler P, Saumon G (1985) Intermittent positive pressure hyperventilation with high inflation pressures produces pulmonary microvascular injury in rats. Am Rev Respir Dis 132:880

Dreyfuss D, Basset G, Soler P, Saumon G (1986) Permeability pulmonary edema due to ventilation with high peak pressure is related to changes in volume, not in pressure. Am Rev Respir Dis 133:A 266

Faridy EE (1977) Effect of food and water deprivation on surface activity of lungs of rats. J Appl Physiol 12:123

Faridy EE, Permutt S, Riley RL (1966) Effect of ventilation on surface forces in excised dogs'lungs. J Appl Physiol 21:1453

Frumin MJ, Epstein RM, Choen G (1959) Apneic oxygenation in man. Anesthesiology 20:789

Fulheihan S, Wilson R, Pontoppidan H (1976) Effect of mechanical ventilation with end-inspiratory pause on blood gas exchange. Anesth Analg 55:122

Gallagher TJ, Civetta JM, Kirby RR (1978) Terminology update: optimal PEEP. Crit Care Med 6:323

Gattinoni L, Kolobow T, Tomlinson T, White D, Pierce J (1978a) Control of intermittent positive pressure breathing (IPPV) by extracorporeal carbon dioxide removal. Br J Anaesth 50:753

Gattinoni L, Kolobow T, Tomlinson T, Iapichino G, Samaya M, White D, Pierce J (1978b) Low frequency positive pressure ventilation with extracorporeal dioxide removal (LFPPV-ECCO$_2$R): an experimental study. Anesth Analg 57:470

Gattinoni L, Iapichino G, Kolobow T (1979) Hemodynamic, mechanical and renal effects during "apneic oxygenation" with extracorporeal carbon dioxide removal, at different levels of intrapulmonary pressure in lambs. Int J Artif Organs 2:249

Gattinoni L, Agostoni A, Pesenti A, Pelizzola A, Rossi GP, Langer M, Vesconi S, Uziel L, Fox U, Longoni F, Kolobow T, Damia G (1980a) Treatment of acute respiratory failure with low frequency positive pressure ventilation and extracorporeal CO$_2$ removal. Lancet 2:292

Gattinoni L, Agostoni A, Damia G, Cantaluppi D, Bernasconi C, Tarenzi L, Pelizzola A, Rossi GP (1980b) Hemodynamics and renal function during low frequency positive pressure ventilation with extracorporeal carbon dioxide removal. Intensive Care Med 6:155

Gattinoni L, Pesenti A, Kolobow T, Damia G (1983a) A new look at therapy of the adult respiratory distress syndrome: motionless lungs. Int Anesthesiol Clin 21:97

Gattinoni L, Solca M, Pesenti A (1983b) Combined use of artificial lung and kidney in the treatment of terminal acute respiratory distress syndrome. Life Support Syst [Suppl 1] 1:315

Gattinoni L, Pesenti A, Caspani ML, Pelizzola A, Mascheroni D, Marcolin R, Iapichino G, Langer M, Agostoni A, Kolobow T, Melrose DG, Damia G (1984) The role of total static lung compliance in the management of severe ARDS unresponsive to conventional treatment. Intensive Care Med 10:121

Gattinoni L, Marcolin R, Caspani ML, Fumagalli R, Mascheroni D, Pesenti A (1990) Constant mean airways pressure with different patterns of positive pressure breathing during ARDS. Clin Respir Physiol (in press)

Green JF, Sheldon M, Gurtner G (1983) Alveolar to arterial PCO_2 differences. J Appl Physiol 54:349

Greenfield LJ, Ebert PA, Benson DW (1984) Effects of positive pressure ventilation on surface tension properties of lung extracts. Anesthesiology 25:312

Hudson LD (1982) Causes of the adult respiratory distress syndrome: clinical recognition. Clin. Chest Med 3(1):195

Knelson J, Howatt W, de Muth G (1970) Effects of respiratory pattern on alveolar gas exchange. J Appl Physiol 29:328

Knoch M (1989) Treatment of severe ARDS with extracorporeal CO_2 removal. In: Gille JP (ed) Neonatal and adult respiratory failure. Elsevier, Brussels, pp 123–136

Kolobow T, Gattinoni L, Tomlinson T, Pierce J (1977) Control of breathing using an extracorporeal membrane lung. Anesthesiology 46:138

Kolobow T, Gattinoni L, Tomlinson T, Pierce J (1978) An alternative to breathing. J Thorac Cardiovasc Surg 75:261

Kolobow T, Spragg R, Pierce J (1981) Massive pulmonary infarction during total cardiopulmonary bypass in unanesthetized spontaneously breathing lambs. Int J Artif Organs 4:76

Lachmann B, Haendly H, Schultz H, Jonson B (1980) Improved arterial oxygenation, CO_2 elimination, compliance and decreased barotrauma following changes of volume-generated PEEP ventilation with inspiratory/expiratory (I/E) ratio of 1:2 to pressure-generated ventilation with I:E ratio of 4:1 in patients with severe adult respiratory distress syndrome (ARDS). Intensive Care Med 6:64

Lachmann B, Jonson B, Lindroth M, Robertson B (1982) Modes of artificial ventilation in severe respiratory distress syndrome. Crit Care Med 10:724

Lemaire F, Amamou M, Rivara D, Simonneau G, Harf A (1980) Static pulmonary pressure-volume curve in acute respiratory failure (Abstr). Am Rev Respir Dis [Suppl] 121:158

Lemaire F, Harf A, Simmoneau G, Matamis D, Rivara D, Atlan G (1981) Echanges gazeux, courbe statique pression-volume et ventilation en pression positive de fin d'expiration: étude de seize cas d'insuffisance respiratoire aigue de l'adulte. Ann Anesthesiol Fr 5:435

Linton RC, Walter FW, Spoerel WE (1965) Respirator care in a general hospital. a five year survey. Can Anaesth Soc J 12:450

Martin L (1980) Hypoventilation without elevated carbon dioxide tension. Chest 77:720

Mascheroni D, Kolobow T, Fumagalli R, Chen V, Moretti D, Duckold B (1985) Respiratory failure following induced hyperventilation. An experimental study. Crit Care Med 13:322–328

Matamis D, Lemaire F, Harf A, Brun-Buisson C, Ansquer JC, Atlan G (1984) Total respiratory pressure-volume curves in the adult respiratory distress syndrome. Chest 86:58

McClenahan JB, Urtnowski A (1967) Effect of ventilation on surfactant and its turnover rate. J Appl Physiol 23:215

Murray IP, Modell JH, Gallagher TJ, Banner MJ (1984) Titration of PEEP by the arterial minus endtidal carbon dioxide gradient. Chest 85:100

Mutz N, Duma ST, Goldschmied W (1983) Inversed ratio ventilation-PEEP ersatz. Anaesthesist [Suppl] 32:83

Nash G, Blennerhasset JB, Pontoppidan H (1967) Pulmonary lesions associated with oxygen therapy and artificial ventilation. N Engl J Med 276:368

National Heart and Lung Institute (1974) Protocol for extracorporeal support for respiratory insufficiency. Collaborative program. NIH, Bethesda

National Heart and Lung Institute (1979) Extracorporeal support for respiratory insufficiency. A collaborative study in response to request for proposal, NHLI 73–20, p. 6. NIH, Bethesda

Osswald PM, Hartung HJ, Klose R, Spier R (1981) Die Wirkung von verlängerter Inspirationszeit und PEEP auf die Compliance und den Gasaustausch bei der mechanischen Ventilation. Anaesthesist 30:71

Pepe PE, Marini JJ (1982) Occult positive end-expiratory pressure in mechanically ventilated patients with airflow obstruction. Am Rev Respir Dis 126:166

Pesenti A, Pelizzola A, Mascheroni D, Uziel L, Pirovano E, Fox U, Gattinoni L (1981) Low frequency positive pressure ventilation with extracorporeal CO_2 removal (LFPPV-$ECCO_2R$) in acute respiratory failure (ARF): technique. Trans Am Soc Artif Intern Organs 27:263

Pesenti A, Kolobow T, Marcolin R, Riboni A, Rossi S, Romagnoli G, Gattinoni L (1982) A double lumen catheter allowing single vessel cannulation for extracorporeal respiratory assistance. Eur Surg Res 14:119

Pesenti A, Riboni A, Marcolin R, Gattinoni L (1983) Venous admixture ($\dot{Q}va/\dot{Q}$) in ARF patients: effects of PEEP at constant FiO_2. Intensive Care Med 9:307

Pesenti A, Marcolin R, Prato P, Borelli M, Riboni A, Gattinoni L (1990) Mean airways pressure vs positive end-expiratory pressure during mechanical ventilation. Crit Care Med (in press)

Peters J, Radermacher P, Kuntz ME, Rosenbauer A, Breulmann M, Bürrig KF, Hopf HB, Rossaint R, Schulte HD, Olsson P, Falke K (1988) Extracorporeal CO_2 removal with a heparin coated artificial lung. Intensive, Care Med 14:578–584

Petty TL, Fowler AA (1982) Another look at ARDS. Chest 82:98

Petty TL, Newmann JH (1978) Adult respiratory distress syndrome incidence. West J Med 128(5):399

Reynolds EOR (1971) Effect of alterations in mechanical ventilator settings on pulmonary gas exchange for hyaline membrane disease. Arch Dis Child 49:505

Rinaldo JE, Rogers RM (1982) Adult respiratory distress syndrome, changing concepts of lung injury and repair. N Engl J Med 306:900

Safar P (1965) Respiratory therapy. Davis, Philadelphia

Shapiro BA, Cane RD, Harrison RA (1983) Positive end-expiratory pressure in acute lung injury. Chest 83:558

Smith JL (1899) The pathologic effects due to increase of oxygen tension in air breathed. J Physiol 24:19

Suter P, Fairley HB, Isenberg MD (1978) Effect of tidal volume and positive end expiratory pressure on compliance during mechanical ventilation. Chest 73:158

Sykes MK, Lumley J (1969) The effect of varying inspiratory-expiratory ratios on gas exchange during anaesthesia for open-heart surgery. Br J Anaesth 41:374

Thet LA, Alvarez H (1982) Effect of hyperventilation and starvation on rat lung mechanics and surfactant. Am Rev Respir Dis 126:286

Tyler D (1983) Positive end-expiratory pressure: a review. Crit Care med 11:300

Uziel L, Agostoni A, Pirovano E, Sedini I, Pesenti A, Fox U, Gattinoni L, Kolobow T (1982) Hematologic survey during low frequency positive pressure ventilation with extracorporeal CO_2 removal. Trans Am Soc Artif Intern Organs 28:359

Webb HH, Tierney DF (1974) Experimental pulmonary edema due to intermittent positive pressure ventilation with high inflation pressures. Protection by positive end-expiratory pressures. Am Rev Respir Dis 110:556

Wyszogrodski I, Kyei-Aboagye K, Taeusch HW, et al. (1975) Surfactant inactivation by hyperventilation: conservation of end-expiratory pressure J Appl Physiol 38:461

Zapol WM, Snider MT, Hill JD, Fallat RJ, Bartlett RH, Edmunds LH, Morris AH, Pierce EC, Thomas AN, Proctor HJ, Drinker PA, Pratt PC, Bagniewsky A, Miller RG (1979) Extracorporeal membrane oxygenation in severe acute respiratory failure. JAMA 242:2193

Inverse Ratio Ventilation with Pressure Control

J. B. Andersen

Recent interest in newer ventilatory support modes has been stimulated by the fact that the only thing we can offer the patient with severe acute respiratory failure (ARF) is to buy time and allow the lung to heal by itself. The mortality from acute adult respiratory distress syndrome (ARDS) has changed little since the first description in 1967 by Ashbaugh et al. However, there seems to be mounting evidence that high peak pressures (P_{peak}) and high fractions of inspired oxygen (FiO_2) should be avoided as this would add further injury to an already compromised lung (Taghizadeh and Reynolds 1976; Kolobow et al. 1987; Denek and Fanburg 1980; Pratt et al. 1979).

One of the new ventilatory support modes is pressure controlled inverse ratio ventilation (IRV). This was first described by Reynolds (1971) looking at different ventilatory strategies in the neonate with hyaline membrane disease. He concluded that the use of a very long inspiratory phase reduced intrapulmonary shunting and caused a marked increase in PaO_2. In addtion ventilation could be maintained with the use of a markedly lower P_{peak}. The use of the technique in adults was first suggested by Jonson (1982) and Lachmann et al. (1982) who stressed the importance of an early and sustained inflation. They achieved this by using a decelerating inspiratory flow. Furthermore, they pointed out the importance of maintaining the airway pressures both during inspiration and expiration, first to recruit collapsed lung units and then to prevent recollapse. Most human studies have thus used a combination of IRV and a decelerating inspiratory flow created by using the pressure control mode on the Servo 900 C ventilator (Siemens-Elema, Stockholm, Sweden) according to the principles laid down by Jonson and Lachmann.

Required Technology

In the last 7 years advances in biomedical engineering have allowed for the development and introduction of various ventilatory modes that allow complete control and manipulation of parameters in a hitherto unknown fashion. This seems to be especially important if one wants to take advantage of the potential benefits of pressure control and IRV. The preset parameters should be constant and easy to monitor. Any changes induced in the lung by this ventilatory mode should quickly be compensated by an appropriate change in inspiratory flow

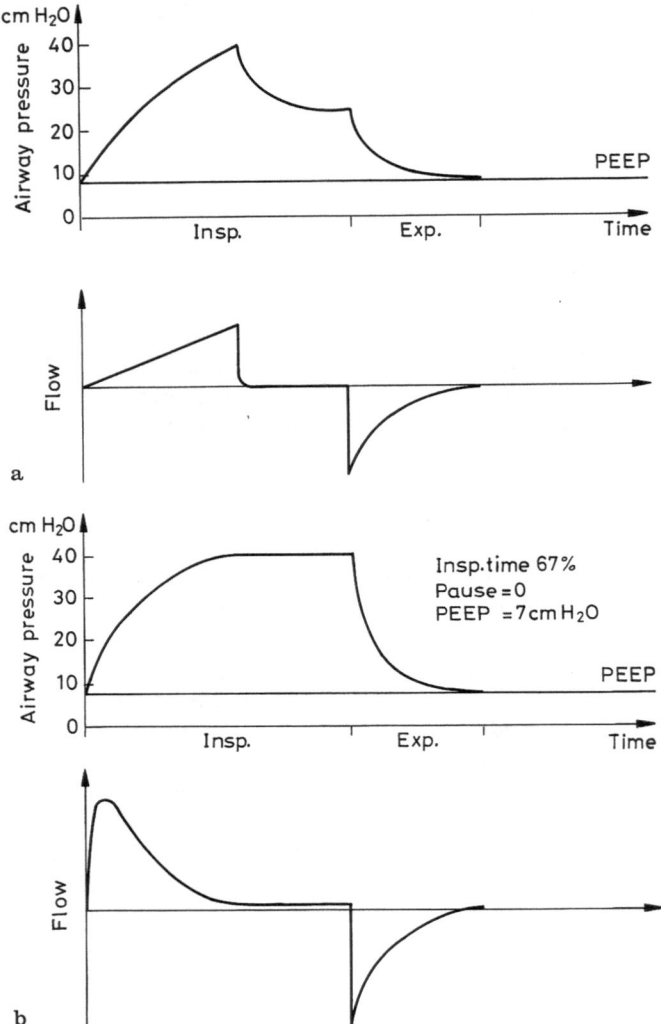

Fig. 1 a, b. Pressure and flow tracings during inspiration and expiration from a traditional pressure controlled respirator (**a**) and from the Servo 900 C (Siemens-Elema, Stockholm, Sweden); (**b**) mode, pressure control with an inspiratory time of 67%

rate. The Servo 900 C ventilator seems to be especially unique in this context. Figure 1 demonstrates the pressure and flow profiles from a conventional pressure control mode ventilator and the Servo 900 C. Clearly the ordinary ventilator fails to maintain the inspiratory pressure required. Furthermore, the ordinary ventilator changes of inspiratory or expiratory times can not be allowed for as compensatory mechanisms inside the ventilator do not exist.

It is important to emphasize that in all successful studies using the newer techniques advantage has been taken of IRV, pressure control, and a decelerating inspiratory flow.

Clinical Documentation

Published studies using IRV with pressure control have included case reports (Lachmann et al. 1982; Gurevitch et al. (1986) and brief reports (Baum et al. 1980; Cole et al. 1984), with only two larger studies (Tharratt et al. 1988; Andersen 1989). No controlled study has been published so far, presumably because of the inherent difficulty in designing such a study in patients with catastrophic lung disease. It would, however, be of considerable interest to perform a study in patients randomized early in their disease process. As usual, endpoints of success differ and in some of the studies patients are not adequately characterized. Lachmann et al. (1982) described six cases of ventilatory failure with dramatic improvement following the shift to IRV with pressure control. The etiology of pulmonary failure varies, however, and the patients are not extensively characterized.

Tharratt et al. (1988) treated 31 patients for various periods of time with IRV and pressure control. Sixteen patients were treated using this mode who had manifested severe respiratory abnormalities requiring high FiO_2s, high PEEP levels and high P_{peak}s. From this study it was concluded that IRV with pressure control can be successfully implemented in critically ill patients for prolonged periods of time with a resulting significant improvement in oxygenation at lower minute volume, P_{peak}, and PEEP requirements. No changes were observed in mean hemodynamic pressures in their patients.

Andersen (1989) treated 105 patients with severe acute respiratory failure all failing to respond to conventional ventilatory support. The patients were well characterized and fulfilled strict criteria including "an adequate cardiac output" to maintain peripheral oxygen delivery. The initial endpoint was to reduce the FiO_2 below 0.6 and the P_{peak} below 50 cm H_2O. In 67 patients in 78 interventions the change to IRV with pressure control was successful. The FiO_2 could be reduced from a median of 1.00 with a range of 0.85–1.00 to a median of 0.45 with a range of 0.35–0.60. This was achieved within a median of 180 min (range, 60–420 min). P_{peak} could be reduced from a median of 70 cm H_2O with a range of 65–85 to a median of 44 cm H_2O with a range of 37–50. This reduction was immediate upon initial adjustments of the ventilatory settings.

It is emphasized that in most patients during the evolution of the disease the ventilatory settings were adjusted on an hourly or daily basis according to need. In 28 interventions an I:E of 2:1 was used, in 40 an I:E of 3:1, and in 10 an I:E of 4:1. The longest time a patient was ventilated with IRV with pressure control was 28 days. The PEEP setting on the ventilator ranged between 4 and 8 cm H_2O and the auto—PEEP had a median value of 12 cm H_2O with a range of 7–22. Forty-one patients did not alter their cardiac output during the change from conventional to the new ventilatory mode. Sixteen patients increased their cardiac output and ten patients decreased it. The largest decrease was 16%.

Physio- or Pathophysiological Consequences

The main findings following the change from conventional ventilatory support to IRV with pressure control in patients with catastrophic lung disease are the decreases in P_{peak} and FiO_2. If high levels of these variables contribute to further lung injury then it is conceivable that such a reduction is warranted.

This new ventilatory support mode has been shown to give a better ventilation to perfusion match with a lower intrapulmonary shunt and dead space. There is substantial evidence indicating that this ventilatory mode creates a higher mean airway pressure although it is debatable whether this can account for the improvement in oxygenation (Cole et al. 1984; Bowe et al. 1983). As dead space decreases, the ventilatory volume demand will decrease and this will tend to move in the same direction as using a lower peak airway pressure. The timing of inspiration and expiration seems to be important. This includes recruiting lung units with a decelerating flow pattern, maintaining the wanted airway pressures during the whole of inspiration and expiration, keeping expiration short, and maintaining the PEEP level. Any creation of auto-PEEP will lead to a nonuniform PEEP distribution (Baum et al. 1980), thereby more efficiently applying the necessary PEEP to lung units with different mechanical properties.

How to Use the Technique

At present the Servo 900 C ventilator is the only one available that can provide the necessary timing control with close monitoring of the essential parameters. The following list suggests how this technique can be implemented:

1. Monitor expired tidal volume.
2. Shift from volume control mode to pressure control mode and adjust inspiratory pressure to provide an almost identical expired tidal volume.
3. Set pause to zero and increase the inspiratory time step by step.
4. When the inspiratory time is at or above 50% check the "auto-PEEP" by stopping the ventilator at end-expiration; adjust the set PEEP accordingly.

Troubleshooting

Example: The inspiratory time of 67% is too short and 80% is too long.
Action: Increase the respiratory frequency.
Example: The $PaCO_2$ falls too low.
Action: Decrease the inspiratory pressure and check that mean airway pressure is adequate. If it falls increase PEEP or respiratory frequency.

In some centers, pressure and flow tracings are used to adjust the ventilatory settings. This can be helpful, but is not always necessary.

References

Andersen JB (1989) Ventilatory strategy in catastrophic lung disease. Inverse ratio ventilation, IRV and/or combined high frequency ventilation, CHFV. Acta Anaesthesiol Scand [Suppl 91] 33:A15

Ashbaugh DG, Bigelow DB, Petty TL, Levine BE (1967) Acute respiratory distress in adults. Lancet 2:319–323

Baum M, Benzer H, Mutz N, Pauser G, Tonczar L (1980) Inversed ratio ventilation (IRV). Die Rolle des Atemzeitverhältniss in der Beatmung beim ARDS. Anaesthesist 29:592–596

Bowe EA, Bowe RL, Klein EF, Buckwalter JA (1983) CPAP vs PEEP. Mean airway pressure does not determine oxygenation. Anaesthesiology 59:A106

Cole AG, Weller SF, Sykes MK (1984) Inverse ratio ventilation compared with PEEP in adult respiratory failure. Intensive Care Med 10:227–232

Denek SM, Fanburg BL (1980) Normobaric oxygen toxicity of the lung. N Engl J Med 303:76–86

Gurevitch MJ, van Dyke J, Young ES, Jackson K (1986) Improved oxygenation and lower peak airway pressures in severe adult respiratory distress syndrome. Chest 89:211–213

Jonson B (1982) Positive airway pressure: some physical and biological effects. In: Prakash O (ed) Applied physiology in clinical respiratory care. Nijjhoff, Dordrecht, pp 125–139

Kolobow T, Moretti MP, Fumagelli R, Mascheroni D, Prato P, Chen V, et al. (1987) Severe impairment in lung function induced by high peak airway pressures during mechanical ventilation. Am Rev Respir Dis 135:312–315

Lachmann B, Danzman E, Haendly B, Jonson B (1982) Ventilator settings and gas exchange in respiratory distress syndrome. In: Prakash O (ed) Applied physiology in clinical respiratory care. Nijjhoff, Dordrecht, pp 141–176

Pratt PC, Vollmer RT, Shelburne JD (1979) Pulmonary morphology in a multihospital collaborative extracorporal membrane oxygenation project. Light microscopy. Am J Pathol 95:191–214

Reynolds EOR (1971) Effect of alterations in mechanical ventilatory settings on pulmonary gas exchange in hyaline membrane disease. Arch Dis Child 46:152–159

Taghizadeh A, Reynolds EOR (1976) Pathogenesis of bronchopulmonary dysplasia following hyaline membrane disease. Am J Pathol 82:241–26

Tharratt RS, Allen RP, Albertson TE (1988) Pressure controlled inverse ratio ventilation in severe adult respiratory failure. Chest 94:755–762

Airway Pressure Release Ventilation

J. Räsänen

Traditional mechanical ventilation effects inflation of the lungs by increasing airway pressure above the ambient. Positive pressure lung inflation reverses the physiological variations in airway and intrathoracic pressure that occur during a normal spontaneous respiratory cycle. Such a fundamental alteration in cardiopulmonary mechanics frequently leads to complications and therapeutic compromise (Montgomery et al. 1985). High airway and intrathoracic pressure during positive pressure breaths does not allow adequate restoration of functional residual capacity with the use of continuous positive airway pressure (CPAP) and, consequently, prevents optimization of gas exchange and lung mechanics (Katz and Marks 1985; Kirby et al. 1975). Increased work of spontaneous breathing and impaired matching of ventilation and perfusion diminish the efficiency of ventilation, thereby leading to an increase in the requirement for mechanical ventilatory support (Froese and Bryan 1974; Wolff et al. 1986). Even when the ventilator is adjusted carefully, positive pressure ventilation (PPV) will elevate mean intrathoracic pressure and result in cardiovascular compromise in patients with normal or low intravascular volume. Periodic alveolar hypertension may cause barotrauma in compliant areas of the lung, may impair healing of the lung, and may even cause additional iatrogenic damage in the diseased alveoli.

An intensive search for better techniques of artificial ventilation has continued for the past decade. Refinements of positive pressure mechanical ventilation have not resolved the problems, because the basic mechanism, periodic positive pressure inflation of the lungs, remains unchanged. However, the most recent addition to the armamentarium of ventilatory support techniques, airway pressure release ventilation (APRV), represents a novel approach to respiratory support. APRV is based on intermittent decrease, rather than increase, in airway pressure and lung volume. The ensuing effects on cardiopulmonary mechanics differ markedly from those of previously used techniques and, therefore, warrant separate consideration.

Technique of APRV

APRV is designed to augment alveolar ventilation as an adjunct to CPAP therapy (Downs and Stock 1987). A CPAP circuit can be modified to deliver APRV by including a pressure release valve that allows rapid transient release of

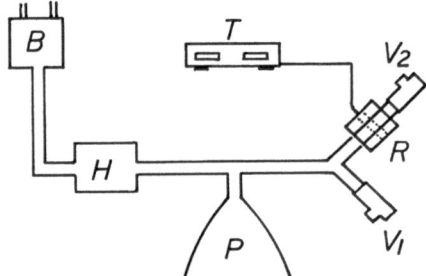

Fig. 1. The APRV circuit. An air-oxygen blender (B) creates a high flow of gas that traverses a humidifier (H) and exits through a threshold resistor valve (V1) creating CPAP when the pressure release valve (R) is open. When the timer (T) opens the pressure release valve, airway pressure and lung volume decrease abruptly to a level determined by a second threshold resistor valve (V2). When the pressure release valve closes, CPAP and lung volume are reestablished, P, patient

circuit pressure from the selected CPAP level to a lower airway pressure (Fig. 1). As the release valve opens and the circuit pressure falls, gas exits the lungs and lung volume decreases by a desired amount below functional residual capacity. When CPAP is reestablished, the lungs are reinflated with fresh gas to the previous volume. Tidal volume of the APRV breath depends on lung compliance, airway resistance, the gradient of pressure release, and the pressure release time. The contribution of the APRV breaths to total minute ventilation and carbon dioxide exchange further depends on the frequency of the APRV breaths. The patient's spontaneous respiration is unimpeded throughout the APRV cycle. The intrathoracic pressure pattern during APRV resembles that recorded during spontaneous breathing with CPAP (Fig. 2).

The application of appropriate CPAP to effect restoration of functional residual capacity is essential for successful use of APRV. Optimization of lung volume with CPAP assures minimum impairment in pulmonary gas exchange, maximum lung compliance, and the highest possible tidal volume for a given APRV pressure release gradient. Improvement in lung mechanics also permits spontaneous breathing with minimal respiratory work between mechanical respiratory cycles. When APRV breaths are added to CPAP, mean airway and intrathoracic pressures decrease, and peak airway pressure remains equal to the level of CPAP (Fig. 2). Therefore, initiation of mechanical ventilation using APRV should neither depress cardiovascular performance nor subject the patient to high airway pressure and the risk of barotrauma.

The pressure release time must be sufficiently long to allow adequate emptying of the lungs, yet sufficiently short not to compromise the efficacy of ventilatory augmentation, or CPAP therapy. A pressure release time of 1.5 s has been used successfully in all previously published studies. The effects of alterations in release times and pressure on gas exchange and alveolar ventilation in various clinical conditions have not been studied in detail.

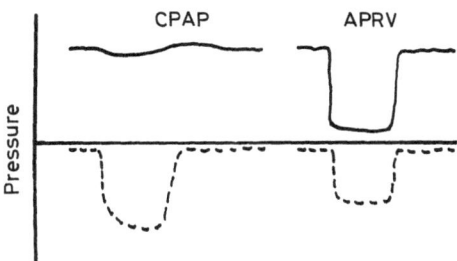

Fig. 2. Changes in airway (*solid line*) and intrathoracic (*dotted line*) pressure during spontaneous breathing with CPAP and during APRV

A ventilator that could deliver APRV is not yet commercially available, nor is APRV an option in any existing mechanical ventilator. Since APRV is designed to be used with spontaneous breathing, the CPAP circuit must offer minimal resistance to spontaneous respiration and a stable airway pressure throughout the respiratory cycle. Therefore, the exhalation valves used to produce the CPAP and the release pressure level must be true threshold resistors with unchanged opening pressure despite alterations in flow. The pressure release valve must effect a sharp, nearly instantaneous drop in airway pressure and minimal resistance to gas flow. This will allow sufficient reduction in lung volume and augmentation of carbon dioxide removal during the APRV cycle.

Respiratory Effects of APRV

Initial experimental and clinical investigations showed that alveolar ventilation and arterial oxygenation can be maintained effectively using APRV (Garner et al. 1988; Räsänen et al. 1988; Stock et al. 1987). Experimental studies comparing APRV and conventional PPV found no significant differences in oxygenation or ventilation in animals with normal lung function when the two ventilatory modalities were delivered using similar airway pressure, tidal volume, and ventilator rate (Stock et al. 1987). However, in dogs with oleic acid-induced lung injury, the use of APRV resulted in significantly lower arterial blood carbon dioxide tension and higher arterial blood oxygen tension compared with PPV. These results suggested that the airway pressure pattern of APRV may favor a more uniform distribution of ventilation than PPV in injured lungs. A study comparing spontaneous breathing, APRV, and PPV using a similar level of CPAP in dogs with oleic acid-induced lung injury, revealed that ventilatory failure and arterial desaturation that existed during spontaneous breathing could be effectively corrected by either APRV or PPV (Räsänen et al. 1988). In this study, arterial blood oxygenation was significantly better and venous admixture lower during PPV. The differences in oxygenation may have reflected mean transpulmonary pressure which, by design, was lower during APRV, or it may have resulted from reduction and redistribution of pulmonary blood flow during PPV. Nevertheless, systemic oxygen delivery was far superior during APRV, because it preserved circulatory function even when ventilation was controlled by hyperventilating the animal.

Peak airway pressure during APRV is 30%–75% of that during PPV (Garner et al. 1988; Räsänen et al. 1988; Stock et al. 1987). Low airway pressure appears to be a consistent major advantage of APRV. The extent of peak airway pressure reduction depends on lung mechanics and on whether APRV and PPV have been adjusted to a similar mean airway pressure or to a similar level of CPAP. Airway pressure levels up to 15 cm H_2O can be maintained safely using a tight-fitting mask in most patients who have intact protective airway reflexes. Since airway pressure during APRV never exceeds the CPAP level, it may be clinically feasible to commence APRV in a patient receiving mask—CPAP therapy without endotracheal intubation. Väisänen et al. have described a patient with myasthenia gravis, in whom postoperative weaning from mechanical ventilation and removal of the endotracheal tube was accomplished successfully by APRV delivered using a mask—CPAP circuit (Jousela et al. 1988).

Circulatory Effects of APRV

The cardiovascular effects of any ventilatory modality are determined primarily by mean intrathoracic pressure and the patient's circulatory status. Therefore, hemodynamic effects of APRV, compared with other types of ventilatory support in a similar experimental or clinical setting, depend on the corresponding levels of intrathoracic pressure. Not surprisingly, no differences in circulatory function have been observed between APRV and PPV in studies that have employed similar levels of mean airway pressure. This has been the case regardless of the presence or absence of acute lung injury or the volume status of the experimental animal or the patient (Halpern et al. 1988; Stock et al. 1987).

However, APRV was originally designed to be used as an adjunct to CPAP therapy. When APRV and PPV are added to existing CPAP therapy, the hemodynamic advantages of APRV become obvious. Increase in the frequency of APRV breaths lowers intrathoracic pressure, augmenting venous blood return. This effect is similar to the hemodynamic response to an increase in the rate or depth of spontaneous breathing. In contrast, enhancement in conventional PPV support increases intrathoracic pressure and reduces venous return, stroke volume, cardiac output, and systemic oxygen delivery. An experimental investigation in dogs with induced lung injury revealed that ventilation could be controlled using APRV, with no depression of stroke volume, cardiac output, and tissue oxygen delivery compared with spontaneous breathing with CPAP (Räsänen et al. 1988). When PPV was used in a similar fashion, stroke volume decreased by 42%, oxygen delivery diminished by 32%, and the oxygen utilization coefficient increased by 33%. Depression in circulatory performance during PPV is commonly seen in clinical practice, and it frequently cannot be avoided. Instead, it must be compensated for by lowering CPAP to a suboptimal level, by infusing large amounts of fluid to augment central blood volume or by using inotropic agents to increase left ventricular contractility. All of these measures are potentially harmful to the patient and complicate therapy considerably. Theoretically, such compensatory support of circulatory function should be required less often, if at all, when APRV is used.

Clinical Role of APRV

Currently APRV is still an experimental technique with clinical applications under investigation. In the first human study of APRV, Garner et al. compared APRV and PPV in patients with mild acute lung injury following cardiopulmonary bypass (Garner et al. 1988). The comparisons were made using similar mean airway pressures for both ventilatory modalities. The results of this study were similar to those obtained in the laboratory under comparable conditions. APRV and PPV provided equally effective ventilation and oxygenation for all patients in the study. Peak airway pressure, however, was significantly reduced during APRV. No hemodynamic differences were detected between the two ventilatory modalities. The patients were weaned successfully from ventilatory support using APRV, and no complications were reported.

Available experimental and clinical data indicate that a marked lowering of peak airway pressure is a major advantage of APRV. Depending on the method of application, mean airway and intrathoracic pressure may be reduced as well. Therefore, use of APRV may lower the incidence of pulmonary barotrauma and the severity of circulatory impairment associated with mechanical ventilatory support. Furthermore, APRV may allow delivery of effective ventilatory support to some patients without endotracheal intubation. Proper evaluation of APRV as a clinical tool awaits controlled investigations in patients with moderate to severe acute respiratory failure of various etiologies.

References

Downs JB, Stock MC (1987) Airway pressure release ventilation: a new concept in ventilatory support. Crit Care Med 15:459–461

Froese AB, Bryan AC (1974) Effects of anesthesia and paralysis on diaphragmatic mechanics in man. Anesthesiology 41:242–255

Garner W, Downs JB, Stock MC, Räsänen J (1988) Airway pressure release ventilation (APRV): a human trial. Chest 94:779–781

Halpren P, Downs JB, Räsänen J (1988) Hemodynamic effects of airway pressure release ventilation and positive pressure ventilation in hypovolemic dogs. Crit Care Med 16:452

Jousela IT, Nikki P, Tahvanainen J (1988) Airway pressure release ventilation by mask— a case report. Crit Care Med 16:1250–1251

Katz JA, Marks JD (1985) Inspiratory work with and without continuous positive airway pressure in patients with acute respiratory failure. Anesthesiology 63:598–607

Kirby RR, Downs JB, Civetta JM, et al. (1975) High level positive end-expiratory pressure (PEEP) in acute respiratory insufficiently. Chest 67:156–163

Montgomery AB, Stager MA, Carrico CJ, Hudson LD (1985) Causes of mortality in
  patients with the adult respiratory distress syndrome. Am Rev Respir Dis 132:485–489
Räsänen J, Downs JB, Stock MC (1988) Cardiovascular effects of conventional positive
  pressure ventilation and airway pressure release ventilation. Chest 93:911–915
Stock MC, Downs JB, Frolicher DA (1987) Airway pressure release ventilation. Crit Care
  Med 15:462–466
Wolff G, Brunner JX, Grädel E (1986) Gas exchange during mechanical ventilation and
  spontaneous breathing. Chest 89:11–17

Monitoring of Mechanical Ventilation

S. Benito

Spectacular progress has been made in the application of new technology in the designing of equipment for mechanical ventilation. This technology has made accurate measurements possible without altering the main function of the ventilator. These improvements have made the equipment not only better on ventilatory support but also infinitely safer. In recent years bioengineers have been studying the equipment we use (Hill and Dolan 1982; Cook and Webster 1982; Ward 1985). The incorporation of measurement systems in ventilators has presented a paradox in that we know more about the pulmonary functional state of a patient when connected to a ventilator than when breathing spontaneously. A simple parameter such as the minute volume is difficult to ascertain continuously in patients with acute respiratory failure who are not connected to a ventilator. Pulmonary compliance is inaccessible initially in such an acute patient in intensive care, but the calculation of both parameters becomes extremely simple once the patient is attached to a ventilator.

In this chapter, we are going to analyze the parameters that are monitored in modern ventilators. The user should know the parameters which are measured by their equipment and how they are measured. These measurements are not a useless sophistication but a guide to the functional state of the patient and they therefore assist treatment.

Monitored Parameters

Airway Pressure

The measurement of airway pressure (Paw) is incorporated in all mechanical ventilators. Originally the most commonly used systems to measure pressures were anaeroids and galvanometers. Now the modern trend is to use electronic transducers displaying the signal value in a digital manner. Airway pressure curves as a function of real time are presented on a fluoroscopic screen which has educational interest.

There are a variety of airway pressures of interest, delivered by all types of ventilators: peak pressure or maximum airway pressure during inflation; inspiratory pause pressure or airway pressure during the inspiratory hold which reflects the alveolar pressure when held long enough (Mancebo et al. 1985);

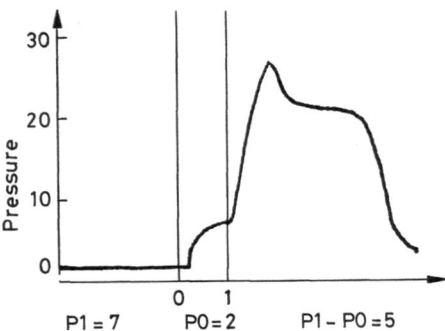

Fig. 1. PEEP measured by occlusion of
the airway at the end of an expiration

expiratory pressure, of great interest because it is the positive end expiratory
pressure (PEEP) value; and in some ventilators (Veolar, Servo C) the mean
pressure during the respiratory cycle. The minimum inspiratory pressure,
although of great value, is not usually displayed but can be calculated on the
displayed image of the pressure curve of a respiratory cycle, and it corresponds to
the pressure needed to open the demand valve. It is an expression of the effort
carried out by the patient to initiate the respiratory cycle. It does not depend on
the sensitivity of the trigger, but rather on the stimulation level of the respiratory
drive (Fernandez et al. 1988). The absolute pressure values displayed by the
ventilator are lower than measured in the patient (Christopher et al. 1985) due to
the pressure drop across the mechanical circuit and depend to a great degree
upon the type of humidifier.

Continuous measurement of airway pressure or, even better, occlusion of
the circuit giving zero flow conditions, provides access to alveolar pressure. When
occlusion occurs at the end of exhalation, before the next cycle begins (Pepe and
Marini 1982) intrinsic PEEP can be measured (Fig. 1). Intrinsic PEEP can be
produced or increased by mechanical ventilation (Caviedes et al. 1986), and it has
effects on the pulmonary mechanics (Rossi et al. 1985).

Tidal Volume

All modern ventilators have some sort of system to measure the tidal volume and
these systems are diverse in their principles and location. In some cases
spirometers are incorporated at the end of the breathing line and measure the
volumes directly while others measure inspiratory flow rates which are then
integrated into volumes.

Although relatively inexpensive the common spirometers are usually
reliable. The hot platinum wire is used by CPU Ohmeda and Eva Draëger, and
the temperature drop above the wire produced by the exhaled gas is proportional
to the gas flow. Deformation of a plate that partially blocks a small hole next to
the expiratory port is used by Servo Siemens. The Engstrom Erica calculates the
time required by a constant gas flow to compress the bag containing the exhaled

gas until it is empty. The Bear system is an ultrasonic sensor placed in the expiratory line. The Bennett 7200 measures volumes by means of a pressure transducer. A solution more similar to the classical respiratory function studies is used by the Pulmosystem and the Veolar and consists of a pneumotacograph placed between the ventilator Y-piece and the endotracheal tube. Besides monitoring the expired tidal volume, a pneumotacograph provides measurements of the inspiratory flow and may be used for regulating the administered gas by means of a feedback loop.

O_2 and CO_2 Concentrations

The measurement of oxygen and carbon dioxide concentrations is now performed by several ventilators. When incorporating an oxygen analyser in a ventilator, the aim is to control the inhaled oxygen fraction (F_iO_2). Due to the physical characteristics of oxygen, three different types of oxygen analysers have been designed. The paramagnetic analysers are based on the magnetic properties of oxygen, which displaces a galvanometer mirror placed in a magnetic field. This is the most commonly used model during anesthesia (Beckman). The galvanic or fuel cell oxygen analyser measures a potential produced by an oxygen sensitive fuel cell. This is the system which is incorporated into most ventilators. The polarographic analyser is similar to the galvanic, using an oxygen electrode, but with a faster response time and thus higher cost. Unfortunately, this type of analyser is unsuitable for use during anesthesia because such an electrode is sensitive to nitrous oxide and this may given misleading results. The most commonly used analyser is the fuel cell, with response time of a few milliseconds. All ventilators are equipped with automatic or manual systems of calibration ranging from air to 100% oxygen. Accuracy is essential for monitoring purposes, the only problem is the battery durability. As long as there is no pressure failure in the medical gas input, the current air-oxygen mixers are very accurate (Baron et al. 1983) and safe although all of them must be tested periodically.

The incorporation of carbon dioxide analysers into ventilators has been an important advance. The basic aim of mechanical ventilation is to eliminate the alveolar gas enriched with CO_2. This situation allows perfect monitoring of the ventilation efficiency. CO_2 analysers use the CO_2 property of absorbing a definitive infra-red wave length. Since the reading is optical, however, it may be disturbed by circuit impurities. Unfortunately, the incorporation of such a device markedly increases the cost of the ventilator. CO_2 analysers are either sidestream (Fig. 2) or mainstream depending on how the gas is sampled. The sidestream systems take the sample in the airway next to the patient. Equipped with a water trap and an aspiration pump, they withdraw a gas sample continuously from the ventilator circuit. The mainstream systems adapt a special piece of equipment with "windows" which are intercalated next to the patient circuit, and thus there is no loss of ventilatory volume. The detector should be warmed to prevent water condensation on the windows. This system induces a slight increases in the dead space of the instrument. Calibration is easier with the sidestream systems.

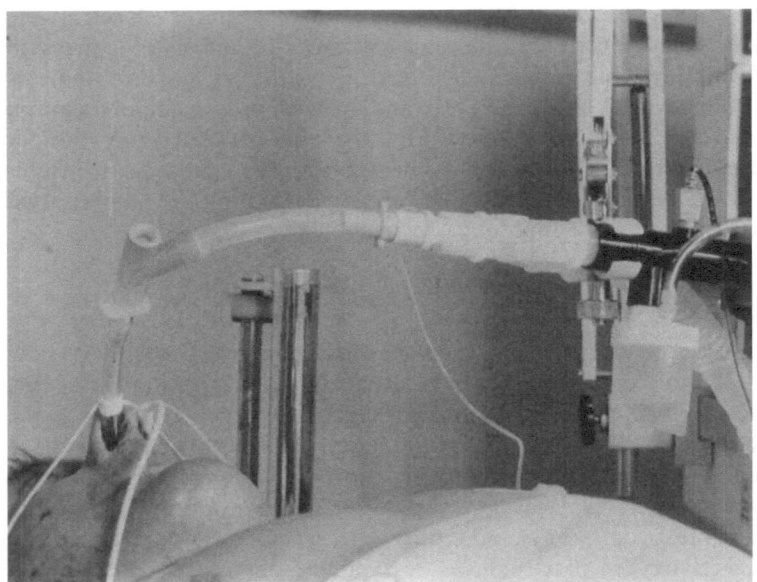

Fig. 2. Sidestream CO_2 analyser (CPU 1)

Capnography is the continuous measurement of the concentration or partial pressure of CO_2 in the Y-piece (Fig. 3). The value of the measurement of CO_2 at the end of expiration (end-tidal, $P_{ET}CO_2$) is related to the $PaCO_2$. Although of some interest when using controlled mechanical ventilation, capnography is useful when using one of the partial support techniques for spontaneous breathing. Monitoring of $P_{ET}CO_2$ allows quick detection of hypoventilation, hyperventilation, apnea, or periodic ventilation (Lemaire 1987). It may also help in selecting the ventilatory parameters, as in a patient with chronic obstructive

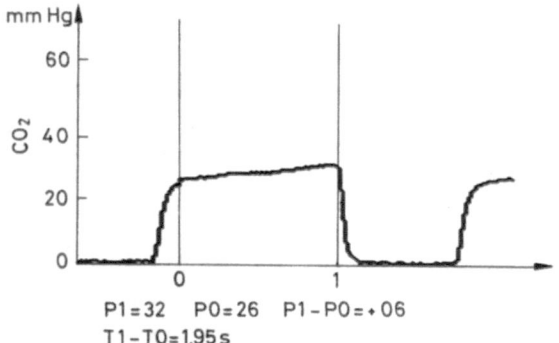

Fig. 3. Capnography

pulmonary disease (COPD) retaining carbon dioxide where $PaCO_2$ must be decreased slowly. The baseline of the capnogram during inspiration should return to zero, thus confirming the arrival of fresh air from the ventilator. An inspiratory value of a few mmHg of $PaCO_2$ indicates rebreathing or some other dysfunction.

Although a physiological gradient exists between the $PaCO_2$ and the $P_{ET}CO_2$, it is increased in many pulmonary diseases and particularly during mechanical ventilation (Bendixen et al. 1965). It is usually stable in the same patient with the same ventilator parameters and continuous monitoring can be used having established baseline arterial blood gas measurements for comparison (Perrin et al. 1983). The gradient $PaCO_2$-$P_{ET}CO_2$ is influenced by dead space, alterations in ventilation-perfusion, and the Haldane effect in ventilated zones. Decrease in the gradient is an expression of better alveolar ventilation and we have demonstrated its value as a predictor of an effective PEEP (Murray et al. 1984; Blanch et al. 1987).

Calculated Respiratory Parameters

Frequency, Spontaneous Ventilation

Methods using partial ventilatory support modes—including intermittent mandatory ventilation (IMV), mandatory minute ventilation (MMV), and pressure support (PS)—demand that the spontaneous respiratory rate and minute ventilation of the patient be monitored carefully. The ventilator may detect the spontaneous respiratory rate of the patient separately (Veolar, Erica, 7200), while other ventilators indicate the total frequency (spontaneous plus machine); CPU, Bear, Servo, Erica, Pulmosystem). The efficiency of the ventilatory performance of the patient is also assessed by monitoring the spontaneous tidal volume (V_T). Some ventilators (Erica, CPU, 7200) measure the patient's spontaneous minute ventilation or measure the machine ventilation as a percentage of total ventilation (EVA). This measurement is especially useful during the weaning period. Monitoring of minute ventilation is obviously crucial for the ventilators providing the MMV mode.

Compliance

The lung pressure/volume relationship is the most commonly used (Goldenheim and Kazemi 1984). The first description of reduced lung compliance in patients with acute respiratory distress syndrome (ARDS) during mechanical ventilation was reported by Falke et al. (1972). Soon after that, Suter et al. (1971) measured the quasistatic thoracopulmonary compliance by dividing the tidal volume by the pressure difference between a long inspiratory pause and the end of the exhalation ($\Delta V/\Delta P$). The Siemens compliance calculator (Janson et al. 1975) was designed to provide breath by breath dynamic compliance values using the same

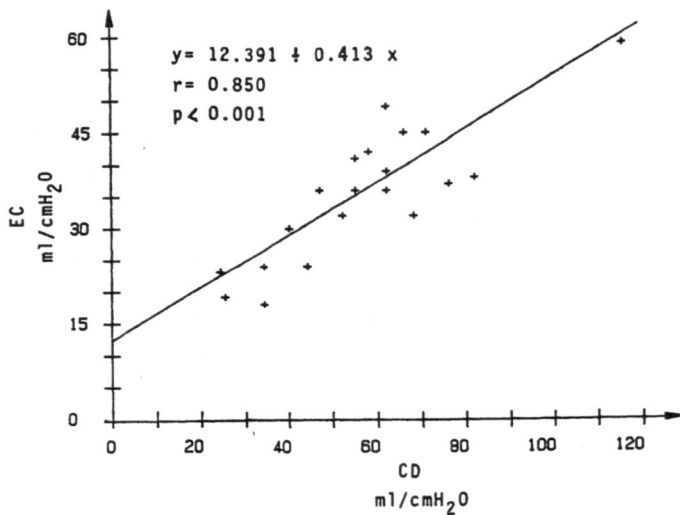

Fig. 4. Linear relationship between quasistatic compliance (EC) and static thoracopulmonary compliance (CD)

procedure. Modern ventilators frequently incorporate an automatic lung compliance measurement device.

Thoracopulmonary compliance is modified by the duration of the inspiratory pause, the lung volume, the level of positive end expiratory pressure (PEEP), and the tidal volume (Suter et al. 1978). For this reason, some ventilators correct the compliance measurement by means of a fixed tidal volume and inspiratory pause (Pulmosystem) or more simply by means of a prolonged inspiratory hold of 1 s (CPU, Veolar, 7200).

We demonstrated that quasistatic compliance shows a linear relationship (Mancebo et al. 1985). to the static thoracopulmonary compliance, measured by tracing the pressure-volume loop (Matamis et al. 1984) (Fig. 4). Dynamic compliance values (in the formula $\Delta V/Pinsp-Pexp$, where Pinsp is the peak inspiratory pressure) exhibit a systematic difference from quasistatic values and are strongly dependent on the flow used. Continuous measurement of pulmonary compliance not only indicates alterations of lung distensibility due to atelectasis or increase in lung water, but it is also sensitive to any endotracheal tube obstruction or displacement, and presence of mucus, bronchospasm, or pneumothorax. Automatic measurement of compliance must take into account the level of auto-PEEP.

Resistance

The airway flow resistance (Raw) is another useful parameter to monitor during mechanical ventilation. This measurement reflects the inspiratory flow resistances of the combination of the patient and the mechanical ventilator. Raw is calculated by dividing the difference between the inspiratory peak pressure and the inspiratory pause pressure by the flow ($\Delta P/\Delta \dot{V}$). The result is given in cm $H_2O \cdot l/s$. In some ventilators, the calculation is corrected for the ventilator resistance. This measurement is not used frequently because many factors may influence it, such as tracheal tube size, circuit impedance, flow wave form, and acceleration. However, any change in the airway resistance of the patient, with no change in the ventilator settings, can be useful as an evaluation of response to treatment.

Carbon Dioxide Production and Dead Space

The incorporation of a CO_2 analyser in some ventilators (EVA, Erica) gives access to carbon dioxide production ($\dot{V}CO_2$), and dead space (V_D/V_T). The information necessary to calculate both the $\dot{V}CO_2$ and the V_D are the minute ventilation and the CO_2 concentration, according to:

$$\dot{V}CO_2 = (F_{\bar{E}}CO_2 \times V_E), \qquad V_D/V_T = \left(1 - \frac{F_{\bar{E}}CO_2}{F_ACO_2}\right).$$

Where $F_{\bar{E}}CO_2$ is the mean expired fraction of CO_2. It is easy to measure the F_ACO_2, or to estimate it from $F_{ET}CO_2$. Conversely $F_{\bar{E}}CO_2$ is measured from $F_{\bar{E}}CO_2$–V_T integration, or after mixing the expired gas in a special box. From $F_{\bar{E}}CO_2$ and $F_{ET}CO_2$, microprocessors can measure V_D, according to the Bohr formula, and $V_D$aw (Fletcher 1985). Knowing V_D can help adjust the V_T and the respiratory frequency of the ventilator (Fletcher and Jonson 1984). Knowing $\dot{V}CO_2$ can help in checking the efficiency of intentional hypoventilation (Dairoli and Perret 1984) or in control of adequate nutrition of the ventilated patient (Laaban et al. 1985).

Display of the Monitored Parameters

Spectacular displays of the parameters monitored by modern ventilators are now available. The old galvanometers, difficult to read, are disappearing and are being replaced by better systems such as digital readouts, bar diagrams, or graphic recorders in real time.

The digital system of liquid quartz gives numerical values for the monitored parameters breath by breath, or the average of several breaths. It allows a display at a distance and provides a more accurate reading (Fig. 5). Bar diagrams (Fig. 6) give a quicker and intuitive impression of the patient's respiratory condition. Once they are familiar with these methods the nursing staff are able to improve control over the ventilated patient.

Incorporation of fluoroscopic screens provides more information about the patient's functional state without the necessity of introducing an external

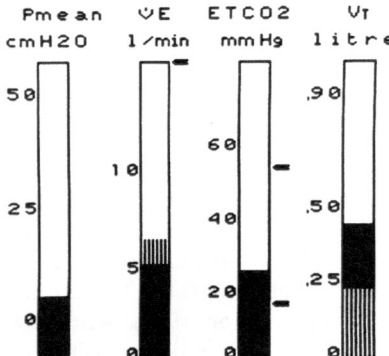

ETCO2 mmHg	32 ⁴¹ ₁₈	F O2	.33 ¹⁹ ₂₅
PPeak cmH2O	36 ⁵⁰	PexP cmH2O	7 ⁷ ₅
PPlat cmH2O	26 :	Pmean cmH2O	10 :
VE l/min	9.8 ²¹ ₆₇	VEspon l/min	.0 :
VT litre	.70 :	VTspon litre	-- :
fmach c/min	14 :	ftot c/min	14 ⁶⁵
C ml/cmH2O	40 :	R cmH2O/l/s	20 ⁹⁹

Fig. 5. Digital system for monitored parameters

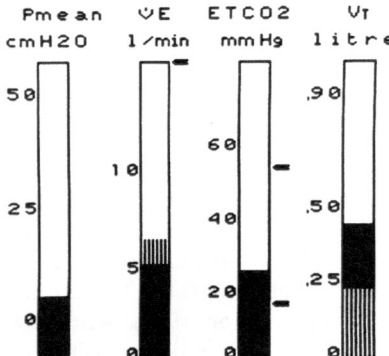

Fig. 6. Bar diagrams

recorder. The potential to freeze any parameter on the screen (like the airway pressure or the exhaled CO_2), allows sophisticated calculations (CPU monitor) to be performed. Widening images, taking reference points, and using bars that take automatic measurements on curve intersection points are additional possibilities offered by the CPU monitor. In this manner, the ventilator is not only a therapeutic tool, it also provides an accurate system of physiological measurements.

One of the extra dimensions of the microprocessors is their memory capacity. This allows recall of how the patient behaved in previous hours, during the day or night, and the evolution of some parameters during treatment. In the newest ventilators, trends of all monitored parameters are depicted (Fig. 7). By means of a screen display or through an interface (RS 232 C) connected to any type of computer, a printer can give these trends over a relatively prolonged period of time.

All these facilities give our patients better overall supervision and provide much better security. The combination of modern monitoring and partial

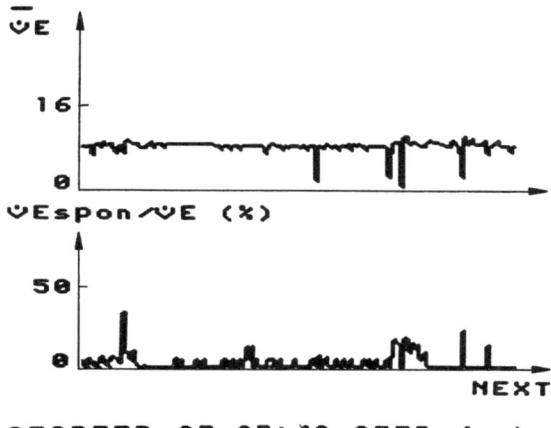

Fig. 7. Trends of $\dot{V}_E$ and percentual relationship between spontaneous ventilation and $\dot{V}_E$

ventilatory support—synchronized intermittent mandatory ventilation (SIMV), continuous positive airway pressure (CPAP), mandatory minute ventilation (MMV), and inspiratory pressure support (IPS)—allows prolonged periods of spontaneous breathing in patients with limited ventilatory reserve under conditions of optimal safety.

Future

The spontaneous ventilatory performance and ventilatory effectiveness of the patient can be assessed by the ventilatory pattern (V_T/T_I and T_I/T_{TOT}) (Younes and Remmers 1981). The measurement of these parameters, with any change over a period of time, are crucial in patients with partial ventilatory support. Manual calculation of F, V_T, V_T/T_I, and T_I/T_{TOT} from strip-chart recording is time consuming and does not give results in real time. However, all these parameters can be easily obtained from any computerized monitoring (Canet et al. 1985).

Inspiratory muscle strength may be assessed by the maximal negative airway pressure (MIP). As all ventilators have a pressure transducer, closure of the inspiratory circuit for 15–20 s (the time recommended for MIP measure standardization) will provide a measurement of MIP in patients undergoing mechanical ventilation (Marini et al. 1980). Measurement of the airway pressure at 100 ms after the beginning of the inspiratory effort of the patient gives a measurement of $P_{0.1}$, which is a good indicator of the activity of the central respiratory drive (Fernandez et al. 1988).

More complicated modifications will allow a more sophisticated investigation of the pulmonary mechanics. A system generating a low continuous flow (Mankikian et al. 1982) could measure the thoracopulmonary pressure-volume curve of the patient together with much more additional information (Matamis et al. 1984). The addition of a SF_6 analyzer gives measurement of the functional residual capacity of mechanically ventilated patients (Jonmarker et al. 1985). Some ventilators are provided with metabolic calculators which give a continuous measurement of $\dot{V}O_2$ and $\dot{V}CO_2$ (Bredbacka et al. 1984).

References

Baron JF, Rieuf P, Herigault R, Lemaire F (1983) Contamination d'un circuit d'oxygène par de l'air comprimé. Ann Fr Anesth Reanim 2:428–430

Bendixen HH, Egbert LD, Hedley-Whyte J, Laver MB, Pontoppidan H (1965) Respiratory care. Mosby S Louis, 72

Blanch L, Fernandez R, Benito S, Mancebo J, Net A (1987) Effect of PEEP on the arterial-end-tidal carbon dioxide gradient. Chest 92:451–454

Bredbacka S, Kawachi S, Norlander O, Kirk B (1984) Gas exchange during ventilator treatment: a validation of a computerized technique and its comparison with the Douglas bag method. Acta Anaesthesiol Scand 28:462–468

Canet J, Viñas J, Navajas D, Casan P, Sanchis J (1985) Variability of the breathing pattern in normals at rest. Bull Eur Physiopathol Respir 21:27A

Caviedes I, Benito S, Mancebo J, Net A (1986) The effect of intrinsic positive end-expiratory pressure on respiratory compliance. Crit Care Med 14:947–949

Christopher K, Neff T, Bowmann J, Eberle D, Irvin C, Good J (1985) Demand and continuous flow intermittent mandatory ventilation systems. Chest 87:625–630

Cook AM, Webster JG (1982) Therapeutic medical devices. Application and design. Prentice-Hall, Englewood Cliffs

Dairoli R, Perret C (1984) Mechanical controlled hypoventilation in status asthmaticus. Am Rev Respir Dis 129:385–387

Falke K, Pontoppidan H, Kumar A, Leith DE, Geffin B, Laver MB (1972) Ventilation with end-expiratory pressure in acute lung disease. J Clin Invest 51:2315–2323

Fernandez R, Benito S, Sanchis J, Milic-Emili J, Net A (1988) Inspiratory effort and occlusion pressure in triggered mechanical ventilation. Intensive Care Med 14:650–653

Fletcher R (1985) Dead space, invasive and non-invasive. Br J Anaesth 57:245–249

Fletcher R, Jonson B (1984) Dead space and the single breath test for carbon dioxide during anaesthesia and artificial ventilation. Br J Anaesth 56:109–119

Goldenheim PD, Kazemi (1984) Cardiopulmonary monitoring of critically ill patients. N Engl Med 311:717–720

Hill DW, Dolan AM (1982) Intensive care instrumentation. Academic, London

Jonmarker C, Jansson L, Jonson B, Larsson A, Werner O (1985) Measurement of functional residual capacity by sulfur hexafluoride washout. Anesthesiology 63:89–95

Jonson B, Nordstrom L, Olsson SG, Akerback D (1975) Monitoring of ventilation and lung mechanics during automatic ventilation. A new device. Bull Physiopathol Respir 11:729–743

Laaban JP, Lemaire F, Baron JF, Trunet P, Harf A, Bonnet JL, Teisseire B (1985) Influence of caloric intake on the respiratory mode during mandatory minute ventilation. Chest 87:67–72

Lemaire F (1987) Monitorización respiratoria durante la ventilación mecánica. In: Net A, Benito S (eds) Ventilación mecánica. Doyma, Barcelona, p 115

Mancebo J, Calaf N, Benito S (1985) Pulmonary compliance measurement in acute respiratory failure. Crit Care Med 13:589–591

Mankikian B, Lemaire F, Benito S, Brun-Buisson C, Harf A, Maillot JP, Becker J (1982) A new device for measurement of pulmonary pressure-volume curves in patients on mechanical ventilation. Crit Care Med 11:897–901

Marini JJ, Smith TC, Lamb V (1986) Estimation of inspiratory muscle strength in mechanically ventilated patients: the measurement of maximal inspiratory pressure. J Crit Care 1:32–38

Matamis D, Lemaire F, Harf A, Brun-Buisson C, Ansquer JC, Atlan C (1984) Total respiratory pressure-volume curves in the adult respiratory distress syndrome. Chest 86:58–66

Murray IP, Modell JH, Gallagher TJ, Banner MJ (1984) Titration of PEEP by the arterial minus end-tidal carbon dioxide gradient Chest 85:100–104

Pepe PE, Marini JJ (1982) Occult positive end-expiratory pressure in mechanically ventilated patients with airflow obstruction. The auto-PEEP effect. Am Rev Respir Dis 126:166–170

Perrin F, Perrot D, Holzapfel L, Robert D (1983) Simultaneous variations of Pa CO_2 and P_A CO_2 in assisted ventilation. Br J Anaesth 55:525–530

Rossi A, Gothfried SB, Zocchi L, Higgs BD, Lennox S, Calverly PMA, Begin P, Grassino A, Milic-Emili J (1985) Measurement of static compliance of the total respiratory system in patients with acute respiratory failure during mechanical ventilation: the effect of intrinsic PEEP. Am Rev Respir Dis 131:672–677

Suter PM, Fairley HB, Isenberg MD (1971) Optimum end-expiratory airway pressure in patients with acute pulmonary failure. N Engl J Med 292:284–289

Suter PM, Fairley HB, Isenberg MD (1978) Effect of tidal volume and positive end-expiratory pressure on compliance during mechanical ventilation. Chest 73:158–162

Ward CS (1985) Anaesthetic equipment. Bailliere Tindall, London

Younes MK, Remmers JE (1981) Control of tidal volume and respiratory frequency. In: Hornbein TF (ed) Regulation of Breathing. Dekker, New York, pp 621–671 (Lung biology in health and disease, vol 17)

Weaning

F. Lemaire and J. L. Meakins

Difficulties in weaning patients from respiratory support are now commonplace in most intensive care units (ICUs) and have only recently been described as a major issue. Weaning failure rates in several large series about 10% (Sporn and Morganroth 1988; Table 1). However, in some risk groups—mainly those with chronic obstructive pulmonary disease (COPD)—failure rates may reach 50% (Pourriat et al. 1986). In a recent prospective study, we identified those patients who could not be weaned. In 1987, 20% of 600 patients mechanically ventilated for more than 24 h in our unit had a weaning period of longer than 3 days (from 3 days to 2 months). These patients had COPD, stroke, paralysis or weakness of respiratory muscles (Guillain-Barré syndrome, myasthenia gravis, myopathy), complications of surgery (Abdominal and cardiac), or, simply, they had been ventilated for a prolonged period of time. These "non-weaners" appeared older (average age, 74 years for the COPD group), and many had a history of left heart disease alone or as a contributing factor. These nonweanable patients are not the majority but represent an important subgroup of ICU patients who cannot be discharged, who require ventilatory support, often for months, and who are a burden upon the morale of doctors and nurses, as well as a drain upon the budget. The newer partial ventilatory support systems have been designed specifically for these patients.

Physiology of Weaning

Recovery of spontaneous breathing is accompanied by two major events, respiratory muscle activation and development of negative intrathoracic pressures.

Respiratory Muscles

The diaphragmatic and intercostal muscle activity comprise only a minor fraction of the total oxygen consumption ($\dot{V}O_2$): the oxygen cost of breathing (measured as the difference in $\dot{V}O_2$ during spontaneous breathing and during full respiratory support with complete muscular relaxation) is usually less than 4% of the total $\dot{V}O_2$ in a normal, resting subject. The oxygen cost of breathing is

Table 1. Rates of Weaning Failure

Authors Year	Weaning failure n	(%)	Diagnosis
Sahn and Lakshminarayan (1973)	17/100	17	Postoperative, ARDS, COPD
Hilbermann (1976)	22/124	18	Postoperative, cardiac surgery
Tahvanainen (1983)	9/47	19	ARDS, LVF, Guillain-Barré syndrome
Nett (1984)		9	COPD
Aubier (1986)	5/16	31	COPD
Tobin et al. (1987)	7/17	41	COPD, LVF, flail chest
Pourriat (1987)	19/37	51	COPD
Fernandes (1987)	4/16	25	COPD
Sassoon et al. (1987)	4/16	25	COPD

ARDS, adult acute respiratory distress syndrome; COPD, chronic obstructive pulmonary disease; LVF, left ventricle failure

increased by exercise and, of course, in patients with COPD, mostly during acute exacerbation of their disease.

However, during the weaning trials, the oxygen cost of breathing may reach up to 50% of $\dot{V}O_2$. The cardiac output increases to fulfill these acute oxygen requirements. Indeed, several studies performed on cardiac surgery patients have convincingly demonstrated that the ability to increase the cardiac output is a good predictor of successful weaning. Difficult-to-wean patients had no change or even decreased their cardiac output after ventilator disconnection (Table 1) (Beach et al. 1973; Wolf and Grädel 1975; Delooz 1976; Mathru et al. 1982).

Intrathoracic Pressures

Mechanical ventilation (MV) creates a positive intrathoracic pressure, while spontaneous breathing (SB) provides a negative pleural pressure. When a patient is acutely disconnected from the ventilator and starts breathing spontaneous, the mean pleural pressure shifts from $+5$ to -8 mmHg (Lemaire et al. 1988). This leads to important hemodynamic consequences: the fall in pleural pressure increases the venous return but also increases the left ventricular (LV) afterload, thus reducing systolic stroke volume. It has been shown that a failing LV can be "assisted" by MV (or continuous positive airway pressure, CPAP) (Räsänen et al. 1984). Conversely, acute disconnection from the ventilator may induce severe cardiac dysfunction (Lemaire et al. 1988).

Pathophysiology of Weaning

The sequence of events leading to weaning failure is well known.

Changes in Respiratory Pattern

Respiratory rate (RR) increases markedly, sometimes immediately after disconnection, predicting a rapid weaning failure. Tobin et al. (1986) showed that seven "nonweaners" had a RR of 32 breaths min with a small tidal volume (Vt) (184 ± 23 ml), while successful weaners had a much lower RR (21 ± 3 breaths/min) and higher Vt (358 ± 56 ml). Inspiratory duration (Ti) was, of course, reduced (0.8 s vs 1.41 s), as was the duration of expiration (Te, 1.24 vs 2.48 s), without significant modifications of the duty cycle (Ti/Ttot, with Ttot being total time). This manifests clinically as rapid, shallow breathing which quickly induces:

1. Increased dead-space (Vd/Vt).
2. Alveolar hypoventilation.
   Both of which explain the hypercapnia which rapidly develops, and
3. Increased in the pulmonary shunt ($\dot{Q}s/\dot{Q}t$), due to the augmented cardiac output and reduced alveolar ventilation, thus increasing ventilation/perfusion nonhomogeneity (Gilbert 1974; Lemaire et al. 1988).
4. Decreased Ti, which induces an increased Functional residual capacity (FRC) in COPD patients due to auto-PEEP ("hyperdynamic inflation"), reducing diaphragmatic contractility and increasing the inspiratory (elastic) work of breathing (Pepe and Marini 1982) (see Fig. 1).

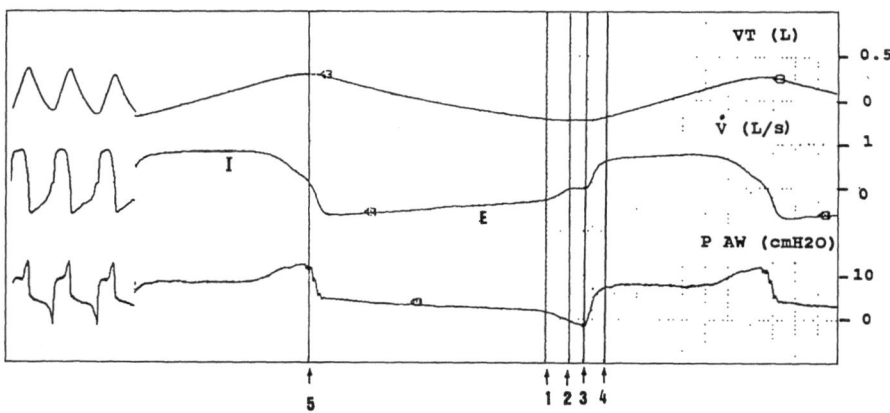

Fig. 1. Auto-PEEP From *top* to *bottom*, curves of tidal volume (Vt), flow ($\dot{v}$), airway pressure (PAW); distance between two vertical lines, 100 millisec. From *5* to *1*: expiration, a slow expiratory flow is continuously present. *1* to *2*, zero-flow period, because the inspiratory valve is not opened yet, airway pressure becomes negative. *3*, due to demand-valve opening, inspiratory flow may increase rapidly. *4*, Plateau of steady positive pressure is reached. Auto-PEEP provides additional inspiratory workload since the first part of inspiratory muscle contraction (*1* to *2*) is wasted (no yield of inspiratory flow)

Asynchronous motion of the rib cage and abdomen (abdominal paradox) has been claimed to indicate diaphragmatic fatigue and to predict unsuccessful weaning (Cohen et al. 1982). Pourriat et al. (1986) examined the respiratory pattern of unweanable patients a few minutes after spontaneous ventilation was resumed. Gastric pressure (Pga) was negative, indicating that the diaphragm did not participate in active inspiration. However, Tobin et al. (1987) have shown that abdominal paradox was found in patients who were ultimately weaned successfully. This is an unresolved problem.

Accessory muscle activation (mainly the sternocleidomastoids) is also a sign that spontaneous breathing will be poorly tolerated.

Respiratory Drive and Occlusion Pressure

Insufficient respiratory drive would, obviously compromise recovery of spontaneous ventilation. It is good clinical practice to start the weaning process only after elimination of sedation and/or treatment of metabolic alkalosis. Not long ago, it was generally assumed that any acute exacerbation of COPD was associated with respiratory drive depression ("central" fatigue). The occlusion pressure ($P_{0.1}$) has recently been used as an index of respiratory derive activity, in ventilated patients and during the weaning phase. Published studies have uniformly reported an increased $P_{0.1}$, suggesting extreme stimulation of the central nervous system (Sassoon et al. 1987). Murciano et al. (1988) measured $P_{0.1}$ of 7 cm H_2O at the beginning of MV of COPD patients. After a few days of respiratory muscle rest, $P_{0.1}$ decreased to less than 3 or 4 cm H_2O in those patients who weaned successfully. Conversely, in the patients who did not, $P_{0.1}$ remained elevated. Since the central fatigue theory was disproved, most weaning failures are now explained by "contractile" muscle fatigue.

Muscle Fatigue and Weaning Failure

Fatigue is difficult to assess in routine, nonresearch practice. Experimental studies have revealed that diaphragmatic fatigue is accompanied by a shift of the power spectrum of the electromyogram (marked by a decrease in the high to low (H/L) ratio) and that it occurs when the H/L ratio is less than 80% of control (Gross et al. 1979). Fatigue may also be diagnosed when the strength developed by the diaphragm (transdiaphragmatic pressure (Pdi) = gastric pressure minus Peso) during tidal breaths is abnormally close to the maximal strength the patient can develop (Pdi-max). A Pdi/Pdi-max ratio greater than 0.30 predicts imminent diaphragmatic fatigue (Bellemare and Grassino 1982). In unweanable patients, Cohen et al. (1982) showed that a decrease in the H/L ratio was a sign of intolerance of spontaneous breathing, before tachypnea, increase in resting minute ventilation (Ve), abdominal paradox, and/or hypercapnia. Murciano et al. (1988), Pourriat et al. (1986), and Brochard et al. (1988a) have produced similar results. These studies all suggest that diaphragmatic fatigue, at least in COPD patients, explains most weaning failures. This failure is probably

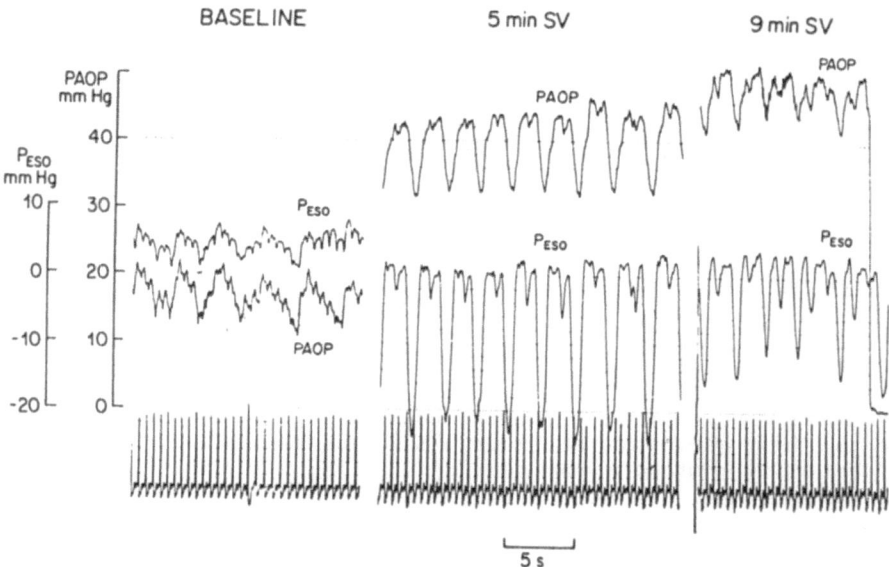

Fig. 2. Acute dysfunction during weaning. During mechanical controlled ventilation (*baseline*), expiratory Peso is $+2$ mmHg, and end expiratory PAOP is 15 mmHg; after a few minutes of spontaneous breathing, mean Peso is decreased (-8 mmHg) and PAOP (exp) is increased to 40 then 50 mmHg. *PAOP*, pulmonary artery occlusion pressure; Peso, esophageal pressure; baseline is mechanical ventilation. SV: spontaneous ventilation, 5 and 9 min after disconnection. (From Lemaire et al. 1988 with permission)

associated with a contribution from malnutrition and the increased work of breathing.

Recently, however, Swartz and Marino (1985) have shown that hypercapnia appeared in seven unweanable patients without any decrease in the force generated (Pdi). The electromyogram assessments used in these studies are only an indirect witness of fatigue; they help identify abnormal breathing patterns known to predict respiratory muscle fatigue (Fig. 2).

Weaning and Left Ventricular Function

Reestablishment of spontaneous breathing requires an increase in cardiac output, and it also induces a sudden drop in pleural pressure. These two factors may unmask or aggravate uncompensated left heart failure. Nikki et al. (1982) and Räsänen et al. (1984) demonstrated that patients ventilated for pulmonary edema resulting from myocardial infarction were easily weaned using CPAP (via an increased intrathoracic pressure). Recently, it was proposed that a failing heart should be supported by positive pressure mechanical ventilation, in accordance with the theory of the Baltimore group (Buda et al. 1979; Pinsky et al. 1983).

In 15 unweanable patients with COPD and a history of left heart disease (mainly ischemic), we showed recently (Lemaire et al. 1988) that disconnection of

Table 2. Hemodynamis of weaning

Author (year)	Type of patients	Weaning	CI		PAOP		SAP		$\dot{V}O_2$	
			CV	SB	CV	SB	CV	SB	CV	SB
Wolff and Gradd (1975)	Postoperative Cardiac	W	2.7	2.9	15	17			137	150
		NW	2.5	2.1	23	24			136	129
Delooz (1976)	Postoperative Cardiac	W	2.3	2.5	6	8	75	85	268	286
		NW	2.2	2.6	10	11	76	84	260	248
Lemaire (1986)	COPD, LVF		2.6	3.4	13	14	72	79	163	178
		NW	2.8	2.8	15	20	80	86	162	151
Fernandes (1987)	COPD	W	4.7	6.3					222	314

W, weaner; NW, nonweaner; CI, cardiac index; PAPO, pulmonary artery occcluded pressure; SAP, systemic arterial pressure; $\dot{V}O_2$ oxygen consumption; CV, controlled ventilation; SB, spontaneous breathing

the ventilator was followed rapidly by acute LV dysfunction with a marked increase in the pulmonary artery occlusion pressure from 7 to 24 mmHg (Table 2). Simultaneously isotopic ventriculography revealed that this LV filling pressure increase was due to an extreme dilatation of the LV or to an acute reduction of LV diastolic compliance because of coronary ischemia or RV interdependence. In more than one-half of these patients, Fournier analysis of kinetic images of the LV disclosed acute segmented dyskinesia, indicating LV ischemia. An 8-day regimen of diuretics and vasodilators ultimately led to a successful weaning in 9 of these 15 patients, even though some of them had been mechanically ventilated for weeks or even months before cardiac dysfunction was discovered and treated.

Acute LV dysfunction may compromise weaning by several mechanisms:

1. Insufficient or no increase in cardiac output.
2. Bronchial edema (cardiac asthma) increasing airway resistance and inspiratory work of breathing.
3. Inadequate or no increase in diaphragmatic blood flow, precluding an increase in respiratory muscle performance (Aubier et al. 1982).

Weaning failure in any patient with a history or signs of LV disease should evoke the diagnosis of LV dysfunction, prompt measurement of pulmonary artery occluded pressure (PAPO) during spontaneous breathing and treatment of cardiac failure, when present.

Strategy of Weaning

Three issues have to be addressed successively:

1. The timing of weaning: global clinical status
2. The ability of the patient to breathe spontaneously
3. The need for a partial ventilatory support

The Moment of Weaning

Obviously, before the weaning process may start, the cause of the acute episode of respiratory failure must be resolved and the patient has to be in a clinically steady state. The identification of appropriate time for weaning must begin with a global clinical assessment. It is unwise to start a weaning trial with a patient who is febrile, in shock, or agitated. This holds true particularly in older, debilitated patients, and those with COPD. If pneumonia was the cause of the acute episode, it must be resolved. Obtundation, encephalopathy, or even coma are not absolute contraindications to weaning from the ventilator provided spontaneous breathing is possible and the cough effective. Extubation, however, may be a problem due to the dangers of aspiration and lack of cooperation. Hypoxemia is rarely a cause per se for postponing weaning, since it is usually corrected by increasing the FiO_2 (Table 3).

Weaning Criteria

Many criteria have been proposed to predict the success of a weaning trial (Table 4). These criteria assess the patient's performance but do not measure the effort involved. Tidal volume (Vt), vital capacity (VC), and minute ventilation indicate minimal resting values. Resting minute ventilation (Ve) needs to be less than 10 l/min, but the patient must be able to double it. Maximal negative

Table 3. Requirements for initiation of weaning

Start weaning only after correction of:
- Metabolic alkalosis (diuretics, bicarbonate infusion, gastrointestinal aspiration
- Sedation (ongoing or recently interrupted)
- Encephalopathy, agitation, coma
- Extreme and/or chronic denutrition
- Fever, sepsis, septic shock
- Hemodynamic instability (shock from any cause, arrythmia, cardiac failure)
- Electrolytic disturbance (low plasma levels of Na, K, phosphorus, Ca)
- Excessive caloric intake ($\leqslant 3000$ kcal/day)
- Untreated (or uncured) acute respiratory disease (mainly bacterial pneumonia, community or nosocomial, bronchospasm, pulmonary edema)

Speed up weaning in the presence of:
- Massive bronchopleural air leak—only negative pressure inspiration may suppress it

Table 4. Usual weaning predictors

Criterion	Value
Tidal volume (Vt)	> 5 ml/kg
Vital capacity (VC)	> 10–15 ml/kg
Respiratory rate (RR)	< 35/min
Resting minute ventilation	< 10 breaths/min
Maximal minute ventilation	Double resting values
Maximal negative inspiratory force	> -25–30 cm H_2O
Occlusion pressure ($P_{0.1}$)	< 7 cm H_2O
PaO_2 ($FiO_2 < 0.4$)	> 60 mmHg
$P(A\text{-}a)O_2$ (FiO_2 1)	< 300 mmHg
$\dot{Q}s/\dot{Q}t$	$< 10\%$–20%
pH	> 7.30
Vd/Vt	< 0.55–0.60
$PaCO_2$ increase after disconnection	$\leqslant 8$ mmHg

inspiratory (MNI) pressure developed against an obstructed tracheal tube should be higher than -25 or -30 cm H_2O. Sahn and Lakshminarayan (1973) studied the predictive value of these latter two criteria in a group of 100 patients during weaning. Seventy-six patients met them and weaned successfully: 24 were unable to double their minute ventilation, and only seven were ultimately weaned. In an earlier study, Browne et al. (1972) established the value of the VC and the maximum negative inspiratory force in a group of 25 patients who had weaned successfully for varying periods of time. Weaning was obtained once MNI pressure was -34 cm H_2O and VC 16 ml/kg body weight. Tobin et al. (1986a) reported on the negative predictive value of tachpnea occurring immediately after the beginning of spontaneous breathing.

The major interest of these measurement is that they can be obtained routinely at the bedside. Minute ventilation is measured by means of one of the numerous commercially available spirometers. MNI pressure is measured at the tracheal tube outlet, when obstructed during a maximal inspiratory effort. The other parameters listed in Table 4 are less commonly used. All indices dealing with oxygenation (PaO_2, PaO_2/FiO_2, $P(A\text{-}a)O_2$, Qs/Qt) are too much influenced by FiO_2. The increase of $PaCO_2$ when the patient is disconnected from the ventilator should be less than 8 mmHg.

Several studies have recently pointed out that all these "classical" criteria are effective only when applied to patients weaning after short-term ventilation, but have a poor, if any, predictive value after prolonged respiratory support. Morganroth et al. (1984) showed in these patients that general clinical indices, based upon temperature, blood pressure, nutritional status, and pulmonary wedge pressure, had much better predictive significance. $P_{0.1}$ (or the pressure measured at the airway 100 m after inspiration against an obstructed tube) is an indicator of respiratory drive much more than is respiratory muscle activity (vide supra). However, an elevated $P_{0.1}$ (more than 6–7 cm H_2O) during acute exacerbations of COPD, and during weaning trials, reveals an exaggerated respiratory drive, and predicts the long-term inability of the patient to breathe successfully on his own.

Fiastro et al. (1982) also demonstrated the failure of the "usual" criteria to predict the success of weaning. In their study successful weaning was correlated with the patient's work of breathing. Additionally, Brochard et al. (1988b) showed that the inspiratory work of breathing in patients during weaning trials was linearly correlated with the oxygen cost of breathing. The work of breathing greater than 6 j/min was also accompanied by evidence of diaphragmatic fatigue (H/L ratio less than 80%). Endurance indices such as the tension time index (Pdi/ Pdi-max × Ti/Ttot) test the ability of the patient to sustain prolonged spontaneous ventilation. Any increase in the tidal diaphragmatic strength (Pdi) compared with the maximum strength the subject can develop and/or lengthening of inspiration duration (Ti) promotes diaphragmatic fatigue.

These objective measurements are reproducible and very useful in identifying the weanable patient. However, they need to be accompanied by clinical observation. To depend upon numbers alone in the face of adverse clinical signs or evolution is to court disaster.

Ventilatory Support During Weaning

When a patient cannot breathe spontaneously for a prolonged period of time using a T-piece system (usually 2 h), ventilatory assistance must be provided in such a way that it will allow respiratory muscle activity without inducing fatigue. The cost-benefit ratio should then be carefullly weighed: on the one hand, the partial respiratory support—synchronized intermittent mandatory ventilation (SIMV), mandatory minute ventilation (MMV), or inspiratory pressure support (IPS)—guarantees safety (alarms, minimal minute ventilation), but on the other hand, connection of the patient to the ventilator circuit (tubing, limited peak flow, humidifer, demand-valve) increases the work of breathing (Marini et al. 1985b). Marini has shown convincingly that the work of breathing can be increased during assisted breaths (intermittent mandatory ventilation (IMV) (Marini 1988) or assist-controlled (AC) ventilation) (Marini 1985a) when the settings of Vt and flow are inadequate. The probable reasons are the inadequate inspiratory flow waveform delivered by most ventilators and the highly resistive demand valves.

These criticisms have forced most manufacturers to follow the Siemens Company, which has added a slight level of pressure support during all of their "spontaneous" ventilator modes. However, we have shown recently (Beydon et al. 1988) that although small levels of IPS increase the spontaneous Vt effectively, they can aggravate the resistive workload of breathing. This is due to the increased inspiratory flow and added turbulence in the circuit and airways. In fact, relatively high levels of IPS are necessary to suppress all the "added" work: 4–6 cm H_2O in normals and 12–13 in patients with a COPD (Brochard et al.

Table 5. Different modalities of respiratory support used during the weaning process

Modalities	Advantages	Disadvantages	Indications
T-Piece	• Easy, inexpensive • Minimal inrease of WOB	• Close surveillance • spontaneous breaths are not assisted	• All patients, especially COPD and uncomplicated postoperative cases
IMV	• Provides a minimal preset V min • Monitoring of the ventilator needs less clinical surveillance • Flexible: full scale of RR between CV and SB • Reversible: when low frequency of mechanical breaths is ill tolerated, it is easy to increase RR	• ↑ WOB if no associated IPS • Manual alterations of mandatory breaths (Vt and RR) necessary: no automatic (or servocontrolled) adaptation to patient's needs	• All intensive care patients, but not the COPD
A-C (Assist-control)	• Patient determines his own RR • Automatic adaptation of low spontaneous breaths	• Can ↑ WOB • Risk of hyper-VE with respiratory alkalosis	• Postoperative patients • Chiefly USA
MMV	• Access to ventilator monitoring • Safety: provides back-up ventilation	• ↑ WOB (like IMV) • Risk of shallow breathing with alveolar hypoventilation • Does not really adapt to patients needs	• CNS disease (stroke, coma) • Peripheral nerve disease (Guillain-Barré, myasthenia)

Mode	Advantages	Disadvantages	Indications
CPAP • Continuous flow • Demand value	• Decreased WOB • Ventilator monitoring • Monitoring	• No monitoring • ↑ WOB (as IMV, MMV)	• COPD $\Big\}$ antagenize auto-PEEP • ARDS • Postoperative atelectasis • Left ventricle failure
IPS	• ↓ WOB, ↓ O_2 cost breathing • ↓ RR, ↑ VT, ↓ diaphragmatic fatigue • Flexible (level of IPS from 0 to 50 cm H_2O) • May be combined with other modes using SB (IMV, MMV, CPAP)	• Too large Vt and apnea when PAW is too high: need of careful titration of the level of pressure plateau	• Any difficult weaning, especially in COPD patients

WOB, work of breathing; RR, respiratory rate

1988b). Table 5 summarizes the indications and contraindications of all modes of partial support.

The T-Piece. The most traditional way of weaning is to disconnect the patient from the ventilator and attach a humidifier to the tracheal tube outlet. If clinical tolerance is evident and satisfactory and blood gases maintained, the patient is extubated. This procedure is used widely for simple weaning for the post-operative period and in COPD patients, and it is usually effective. Should it fail, however, reintubation is required. Weaning using the T-piece demands close surveillance of the patient who is at risk for developing fatigue, sudden respiratory failure, and cardiac arrest.

IMV and AC Ventilation. Although IMV rapidly became a standard mode of MV, it was originally designed as a weaning tool. Efficiency in that respect was never definitely established. Downs et al. (1974) reduced the total MV period from 38 to 24 h. However, in a critical editorial, Petty (1975) outlined all the flaws of randomization in their study. Similarly, Schachter et al. (1981) claimed recently that introducing IMV in their ICU lengthened the mean duration of ventilatory support from 30 to 60 days. Conversely, applying IMV to patients with flail chest decreased the ventilation time from 19 to 5 days in a study by Cullen et al. (1975).

However, the nature of a difficult weaning process should not be evaluated only by the duration of MV. Safety is at least as important. Nearly all (published) comparisons of different weaning procedures do not pay enough attention to that essential feature. At present, it seems clear that IMV is losing ground to the pressure support ventilation (PSV) mode. The main reason is that IMV is illogical in supplying some mechanical breaths in addition to basically unassisted breaths, while IPS supplements every spontaneous breath in a highly flexible way.

AC ventilation has also been progressively replaced by newer modes, although it used to be, especially in the USA, The mode (par excellence) of

Table 6. Maneuvers in ventilation of patients with adult ARDS

Maneuver	Effect
1. Decrease FiO_2	1. Reduction of O_2 toxicity
2. Return to spontaneous breathing • IMV • Then CPAP	2. Suppression of: • Hemodynamic support • Swan-Ganz catheters • Early preparation for weaning
3. Decrease PEEP level, according to: • Gas exchange, PaO_2, Qs/Qt, $P(a\text{-}A)O_2$ • Total quasistatic compliance • Chest X-ray	3. Reduction of barotrauma
4. Extubation and continuation of CPAP via a face mask	Prevent alveolar collapse

weaning. Basically, it is not flexible enough, since the patient can only control the respiratory rate, and not the Vt.

Mandatory Minute Ventilation (MMV). This mode is safe and useful for patients with one very specific problem: fluctuation in their respiratory drive. Although, at present still underdeveloped, MMV should improve and be more utilized in the near future.

CPAP. This mode also has very specific indications (see Table 6). It has been recently demonstrated that CPAP can safely antagonize auto-PEEP in SB patients (Petrof et al. 1990).

IPS. This is presently the most frequently used mode of ventilation for difficult weaning, chiefly in patients with COPD (Kacmarek 1988).

Special Characteristics of Weaning

Weaning ARDS Patients

Surprisingly enough, this still severe disease is not really a problem during the weaning phase (Table 6). Classically, the control mode was used until complete recovery, PEEP level being gradually decreased to zero. Nowadays, there is a tendency to keep the PEEP level as high as 10–12 cm H_2O and to reintroduce progressively spontaneous breaths (IMV or IPS). Thus, the patient is kept for a few days on CPAP before extubation, followed by a CPAP mask for a short period of time. The rationale for doing so originated in the finding by Feeley et al. (1975) that alveolar instability persisted long after apparent resolution of the acute event. PEEP of 5 cm H_2O applied to 25 patients during weaning after an episode of acute respiratory failure (ARF) markedly reduced the alveolar-arterial oxygen difference and increased VC and inspiratory force. During this period, persisting hypoxemia is easily corrected by FiO_2 increase. This method of weaning can be successfully applied during the initial steps of the disease (florid edema). Later, when interstitial fibrosis has taken place, CPAP may be poorly tolerated.

COPD Patients and Weaning

Patients ventilated for an acute exacerbation of COPD are probably the most difficult to wean (Fig. 3). The entire procedure may last several weeks or, infrequently, even months. These patients share multiple problems including malnutrition, increased bronchial resistance, asynchrony between the diphragm and rib cage, encephalopathy, increased dead space (emphysema), and an associated ischemic heart failure, or any other cause for LV dysfunction.

Table 7 summarizes general rules to be observed in the treatment of COPD. Many of them are just commonsense, such as wait until the end of the acute episode, restoration of a steady state, and the absence of any acute intercurrent

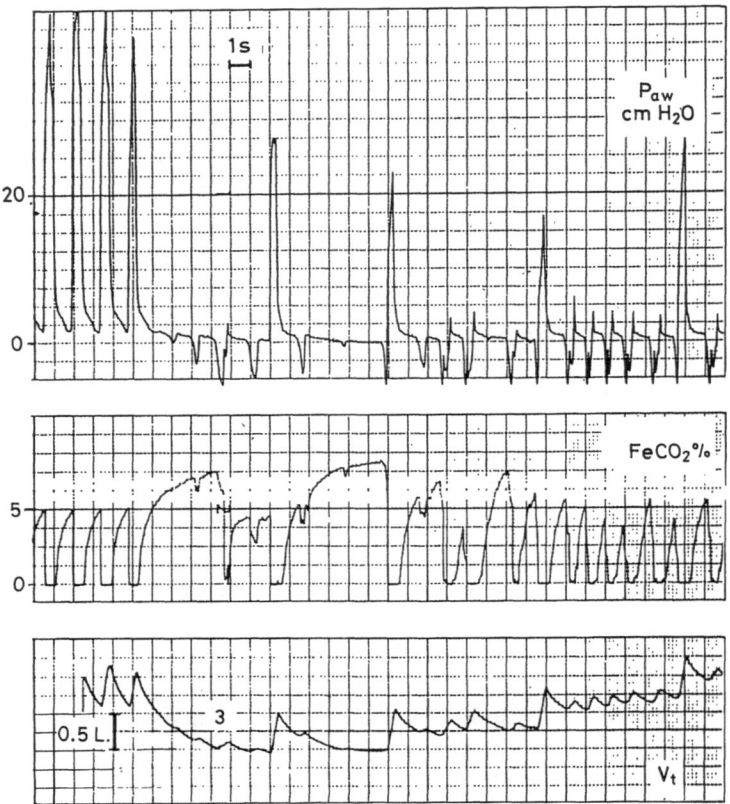

Fig. 3. COPD patient with auto-PEEP. Initially, the patient is ventilated, using a controlled mode, receiving a Vt of 0.5 l. Note that peak PAW reaches 40 cm H_2O. When IMV is initiated, a prolonged expiration ensues, yielding a "trapped" Vt of 1.2 l (auto-PEEP). First spontaneous breaths are inefficient, not providing fresh gas (without CO_2) at the CO_2 sensor. After a few seconds, respiratory rate increases, Vt reaches 0.150 to 0.2 l and $FeCO_2$ is decreased. During IMV, the first spontaneous breath following the mechanical cycle is the weakest, due to enhanced auto-PEEP. *PAW*, peak airway pressure; FeCO, fraction of expired CO_2; *Vt*, tidal volume.

episode. It is also wise to slightly hypoventilate these patients to permit their $PaCO_2$ levels to reach previous levels of hypercarpnia (when they are known), and thus avoid rapid respiratory acidosis after disconnection. The sitting position eases diaphragmatic excursion.

Patients with chronic bronchitis are highly sensitive to an increase in bronchial resistance: bronchospasm must be treated or prevented and secretions carefully suctioned before and during the weaning trial. The inspiratory work of breathing is considerably increased by endotracheal tubes with too small a diameter, insensitive demand valves, or cascade humidifiers, which explains the

Table 7. Summary of rules for weaning a patient with COPD

---

1. Treat the cause of acute exacerbation (pneumothorax, acute bronchitis, pneumonia, pulmonary embolism)
2. Wait until the end of the acute episode
3. Give enteral or parenteral nutrition (but not too much!)
4. Ensure that the patient is in steady state
5. Ensure that $PaCO_2$ is at its "usual" level (can be elevated)
6. To be undertaken after careful tracheobronchial suction
7. To be undertaken after bronchodilatation, if needed
8. Patient should be sitting
9. Diagnose (Swan-Ganz catheterization) and treat (vasodilators, diuretics, inotropes) left ventricle dysfunction unmasked by spontaneous breathing
10. After a brief trial using T-piece, extubate
11. If extubation (or T-piece) fails, use partial ventilatory support (IMV or, more often, IPS): start with a plateau of 25–30 cm H_2O PAW, and then decrease by 2 cm H_2O steps the IPS level, according to blood gases, Vt, and clinical tolerance; extubate when PAW is 10–12 cm H_2O
12. If failure occurs again, attempt:
    - Tracheostomy
    - Short controlled period of T-piece ventilation: 5–10 min every hour
    - Letting patient rest at night, with trials of spontaneous breathing only during day time

---

frequent irrelevance of IMV in these patients. So far, IPS is the only mode really suitable for COPD patients since it has been proved to increase Vt, decrease the respiratory rate, and reduce the "added" work of breathing, as well as the oxygen cost of breathing (Brochard et al. 1988a, b).

Recently, Chopin et al. (1983) proposed MV CO_2, as a new approach to weaning these patients. The ventilator is servo-controlled by the end tidal level of CO_2. When $PetCO_2$ exceeds the preset upper alarm limit (indicating alveolar hypoventilation), the ventilator resumes delivering mechanical cycles, which are interrupted when the lower alarm limit is reached.

Persistant failure after weeks or months leads to permanent tracheostomy, and sometimes to home ventilation.

Weaning and Nutrition

It is beyond the scope of this review to discuss the influence of nutrition on diaphragm muscular mass, and its role in preventing altrophy during MV. In addition, the significance of nutrition in the maintenance of mean body mass and preservation of energy reserves in preparation for weaning, while important but controversial, is also beyond our mandate. This section will discuss only nutritional support during the weaning process.

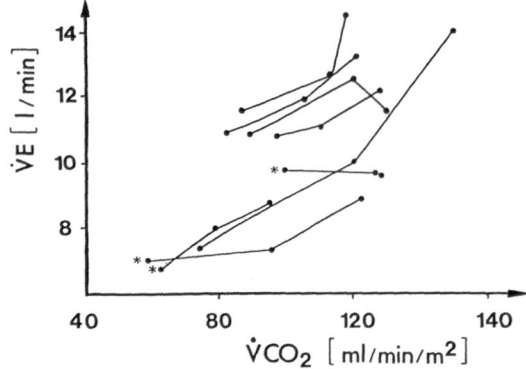

Fig. 4. Relationship between CO_2 production ($\dot{V}CO_2$) and minute ventilation ($\dot{V}E$) in eight patients with MMV. Each patient received three levels of caloric intake. (∗) identify patients with COPD. (From Laaban et al. 1985 with permission)

Do patients need to be fed to be weaned? This is a major issue, without a clear answer at present. An increased level of CO_2 is the main determinant of breathing. Sheep stop breathing when CO_2 levels are lowered and controlled via an extracorporeal circuit (see chapter by Gattinoni et al.). Therefore, any patient during the weaning period should be given some caloric load, to ensure a stimulation of respiratory centers. Bassili and Deitel (1981) compared the rate of weaning in two groups of patients, one receiving 2000–3000 kcal/day, and the other no artificial nutrition (400 kcal/day). Weaning was more successful in the group receiving nutrition: 93% versus 54%. However, one could argue that this study was retrospective and without any form of randomization. We studied the influence of caloric intake on the ability of patients to breathe spontaneously while ventilated by an MMV mode (Fig. 4) (Laaban et al. 1985). When patients received only 400 kcal/day, there was practically no spontaneous breathing and patients were considered to be "unweanable." When caloric intake was increased to 2300, then 3300 kcl/day, the percentage of spontaneous breathing increased to 50% and 82% respectively. Indeed, in these patients, caloric intake improved their likelihood of successful weaning.

Conclusion

Weaning often remains an "exercice de style," an art and science, to paraphrase a recent editorial by J. Milic-Emili, with no magic numbers, no guaranteed predictors, no infallible ventilatory techniques. Conversely, successful weaning is often only achieved after a prolonged period, with the help of patience, good clinical observation, and a comprehensive appreciation of the patient, using repeated assessments of respiratory muscle performance, with understanding, and the wise use of partial ventilatory support modalities.

References

Aubier M, Viires G, Syllie R, Moles N, Roussos C (1982) Respiratory muscle contribution to lactic acidosis in low cardiac output. Am Rev Respir Dis 126:648–652

Bassili HR, Deitel M (1981) Effects of nutritional support on weaning patients of mechanical ventilators. J Parenter Nutr 5:161–163

Beach T, Millen E, Grenvik A (1973) Hemodynamic response to discontinuance of mechanical ventilation. Crit Care Med 1:85–90

Bellemare F, Grassino A (1982) Effects of pressure and timing of contraction on human diaphragm failure. J. Appl Physiol 53:625–647

Beydon L, Chasse M, Harf A, Lemaire F (1988) Inspiratory work of breathing during spontaneous ventilation using demand valves and continuous flow systems. Am Rev Respir Dis 138:300–304

Brochard L, Harf A, Lorino H, Lemaire F (1988a) Inspiratory pressure support prevents diaphagmetic fatigue during weaning from mechanical ventilation. Am Rev Respir Dis 139:513–521

Brochard L, Rua F, Lorino H, Lemaire F, Harf A (1988b) The extra-work of breathing due to endotracheal tube is abolished during inspiratory pressure support breathing. Am Rev Respir Dis [Suppl 2] 137:A64

Browne AGR, Pontoppidan H, Chiang H (1972) Physiological criteria for weaning patients from prolonged artificial ventilation (abstr). Annual Meeting of the American Society of Anesthesiologists, Boston, pp 69–70

Buda AJ, Pinsky MR, Ingels NB, Daughters GT, Stinson EB, Alderman EL (1979) Effect of intrathoracic pressure on left ventricular performance. N Engl J Med 301:453–459

Chopin C, Fourrier F, Chambrin MC (1983) Nouvelle technique de sevrage de l'assistance ventilatoire: ventilation asservie au gaz carbonique. Presse Med 12:495–497

Cohen CA, Zagelbaum G, Gross D, Roussos C, Macklem PT (1982) Clinical manifestations of inspiratory muscle fatigue. Am J Med 73:308–316

Cullen P, Modell JH, Kirby RR, Klein EF, Long W (1975) Treatment of flail chest. Arch Surg 110:1099–1103

Delooz HH (1976) Factor influencing successful discontinuance of mechanical ventilation after open heart surgery: a clinical study of 41 patients. Crit Care Med 4:265–270

Downs JB, Derkins HM, Modell JH (1974) Intermittent mandatory ventilation. Arch Surg 109:519–523

Feeley TW, Saumarez R, Klick JM, McNabb TG, Skillman JJ (1975) Positive-end expiratory pressure in weaning patients from controlled ventilation. Lancet 1:725–728

Fiastro SC, Campbell SC, Shon BY, Habib MP (1982) Comparisons of standard weaning parameters and mechanical work of breathing in mechanically ventilated patients. Am Rev Respir Dis [Suppl 2] 133:A122

Gilbert R (1974) The first few hours off a respirator. Chest 65:152–157

Gross D, Grassino A, Ross WRD, Macklem PT (1979) Electromyogram of diaphragmatic fatigue. J Appl Physiol 46:1–7

KacMarek RM (1988) The role of pressure-support ventilation in reducing the work of breathing. Respir Care 33:99–120

Laaban JP, Lemaire F, Baron JF, Trunet P, Harf A, Bonnet JL, Teisseire B (1985) Influence of caloric intake on the respiratory mode during mandatory minute ventilation. Chest 87:67–72

Lemaire F, Teboul JL, Cinotti L, Guillen G, Abrouk F, Steg G, Macquinmavier I, Zapol WM (1990) Acute left ventricular dysfunction during unsuccessful weaning from mechanical ventilation. Anesthesiology 69:171–179

Marini JJ, Capps JS, Culver BH (1985a) The inspiratory work of breathing during assisted mechanical ventilation. Chest 87:612–618

Marini JJ, Culver BH, Kirk W (1985b) Flow resistance of exhalation valves and positive-end espiratory pressure devices used in mechanical ventilation. Am Rev Respir Dis 131:850–854

Marini JJ, Smith TC, Lamb VJ (1988) External work output and fag generatig during SIMV Am Rev Respir Dis 138:1169–1179

Mathru M, Rao TLK, EL ETR AA, Pifarre R (1982) Hemodynamic response to changes in ventilatory patterns in patients with normal and poor left ventricular reserve. Crit Care Med 10:423–426

Morganroth ML, Morganroth JL, Petty TL (1984) Criteria for weaning from prolonged mechanical ventilation. Arch Intern Med 144:1012–1016

Morganroth ML, Morganroth JL, Petty TL (1984) Criteria for weaning from prolonged mechanical ventilation. Arch Intern Med 144:1012–1016

Murciano D, Bolzkowski J, Lecoguic Y, Milic Emili J, Pariente R, Aubier M (1988) Tracheal occlusion pressure: a simple index to monitor respiratory muscle fatigue during ARF in patients with COPD. Ann Intern Med 108:800–805

Nikki P, Räsänen J, Tahvanainen J, Makeläinen A (1982) Ventilatory pattern in respiratory failure arising from acute myocardial infarction. Crit Care Med 10:75–78

Pepe PE, Marini JJ (1982) Occult positive end expiratory pressure in mechanically ventilated patients with airflow obstruction. Am Rev Respir Dis 126:166–170

Petrof BJ, Legaré M, Goldberg P, Milic-Emili J, Gottfried SB (1990) CPAP reduces work of breathing and dyspnea during weaning from mechanical verification in severe COPD Am Rev Resp Dis 141:281–289

Petty TL (1975) IMV versus IMC (Editorial). Chest 67:630–631

Pinsky MR, Summer WR, Wise RA, Permutt S, Bromberger-Barnea B (1983) Augmentation of cardiac function by elevation of intra-throacic pressure. J Appl Physiol 54:950–955

Pourriat JL, Lamberto C, Hoang P, Fournier JL, Vasseur B (1986) Diaphragmatic fatigue and breathing pattern during weaning from mechanical ventilation in COPD. Chest 90:703–707

Räsänen J, Nikki P, Heikkila J (1984) Acute myocardial infarction complicated by respiratory failure. The effects of mechanical ventilation. Chest 85:21–28

Sahn SA, Lakshminarayan S (1973) Bedside criteria for discontinuation for mechanical ventilation. Chest 63:1002–1005

Sassoon CS, TE TT, Mahutte CK, Light RW (1987) Airway occlusion pressure: an important indicator for successful weaning in patients with EOPD. Am Rev Respir Dis 135:107–113

Schachter EN, Tucker D, Beck GJ (1981) Does intermittent mandatory ventilation accelerate weaning? JAMA 246:1210–1214

Sporn PHS, Morganroth MI (1988) Discontinuation of mechanical ventilation. Clin Chest Med 9:113–126

Swartz MA, Marino PI (1985) Diaphragmatic strength during weaning from mechanical ventilation. Chest 88:736–739

Tobin MJ, Dantzker D (1986) Mechanical ventilation and weaning. In: Dantzker D (ed) Cardiopulmonary critical care. Grune and Stratton, New York, pp 203–262

Tobin MJ, Perez W, Guenther SM, Jemmes BJ, Mador MJ, Allen SJ, Lodato RF, Dantzker DR (1986) The pattern of breathing during successful and unsuccessful trials of weaning from mechanical ventilation. Am Rev Respir Dis 134:1111–1118

Tobin MJ, Perez W, Guenther SM, Lodato RF, Dantzker D (1987) Does rib cage abdominal paradox signify respiratory muscle fatigue? J Appl Physiol 63:851–860

Wolff G, Grädel E (1975) Haemodynamic performance and weaning from mechanical ventilation following open heart surgery. Intensive Care Med 1:99–104

Ventilator Circuits and Their Maintenance

P. Rieuf and P. Tassin

Ventilator equipment maintenance includes cleaning, sterilization, adjustment, servicing, and repair. There are two ways of doing this:

1. All maintenance procedures can be performed by a biomedical central service unit in charge of the ventilators of the whole hospital. The principal problem here is the possible lack of cooperation between the technical and medical staff, leading to what might be called a "technical desert."
2. Maintenance can be carried out between the various ICUs. The biomedical service center does only essential repairs, with or without the assistance of outside after-sales service engineers. In this case, maintenance work is available only if there is a small specialized team responsible for preventive maintenance inside the ICU. Its main responsibilities are to ensure optimal utilization, constant surveillance, detection and correction of minor faults, and instruction of the users.

This is the way to achieve ideal working conditions and to enhance reliability and durability of the equipment. It is obvious that regular servicing is better than expensive repairs and is less costly in the longrun. Both systems working together would be more efficient, but this is difficult to achieve because of the restrictions in personnel.

Ventilator Circuits and Maintenance

First, the composition of the maintenance team must be defined.

The Maintenance Team

In theory, all the intensive care equipment maintenance work can be done by the following staff:

—Nursing assistants for cleaning, assembly, and sterilization
—Nurses for replacement of circuits
—ICU respiratory therapist
—Nurse for day to day supervision
—Physician or anesthesist resident in the ICU

—Biomedical technician
—Biomedical engineer

This specialized team must be responsible for all the maintenance work inside the ICU to ensure that all ventilators are in good working order. The team forms an integral part of patient care and therefore must be properly trained. It is the task of the ICU respiratory therapist to do this and to select nurses and assistant nurses from each unit for training. The maintenance team should work hand in hand with the physiotherapists, and at least one of them should be present all day long. Having been trained to clean, sterilize, and prepare ventilators, the members of the team are also capable of looking after the basic controls of the ventilator and correcting minor faults. They can also advise their colleagues on the use of home device modes and at the same time provide continual instruction (Groupe de Travail sur les Respirateurs de l'Assistance Publique de Paris 1982).

Cleaning, Sterilization, and Preparation Plan

After use, each ventilator must be sent to the cleaning room, where it must be immediately and thoroughly treated. The patient circuit and the expiratory block must be dismantled and cleaned as well as the exterior parts of the ventilator. The flow transducers are disinfected in alcohol and stored in a sterile place. All the respirometers receive the same treatment. Ideally the nurse in charge of the patient using the particular ventilator should do this in order for her to become fully confident in its use and assembly (Chatburn 1989).

When cleaned the ventilator is returned to the preparation room where it is either reassembled or awaits future assembly. All necessary equipment is kept here in sterile containers or covers, so that it can be quickly prepared for use. This room contains a filing cabinet with all the technical and procedural manuals of the various ventilators used which the nurses or technicians can consult. Once assembled the working of the ventilator must be checked and set up for normal use.

Leak tests and alarm tests are carried out. Standard parameter settings are as follows:

—Mode: controlled ventilation, without PEEP
—FiO_2: 0.6
—Frequency: 20 breaths/min
—Minute volume: 12 l/min
—Maximum airway pressure: 60 cm H_2O
—I/E ratio: 1/1.5 (or 1/2)
—Humidifier temperature according to model

When these adjustments have been carried out (Appendix 10.1–10.4), the ventilator is tested on a test lung for 10 min to allow the electronics to warm up. If this check is completed satisfactorily, the refill bag system, when used, can be attached to the humidifier connector. A label indicating the date of the preparation and the name of the person responsible is attached to the ventilator in the pocket provided. Alternatively monthly time-table can be used, listing all the measures carried out on each ventilator. When the ventilator is ready for use it is placed in the awaiting section.

Type of Circuits

Two types of circuit can be used:

1. **Universal simplified circuits.** These consists of two lengths of tubing sufficiently long for connecting the ventilator to the patient, a Y-piece, and an artificial nose which must be polyvalent and easily changeable during ventilation. They must be kept in a place easily accessible to all personnel, since they are simple to use.

2. **Complete circuits.** These should be ready to be fitted to the ventilator and kept in the preparation room, ready to use, sterile and stored, according to the method employed.

The method of sterilization has to be appropriate for the various connectors, the humidifier and accessories, the water traps and the tubes, in order to avoid damage. The different components can be sterilized either separately or assembled, thus making it possible to use them quickly.

When the ethylene oxide system with a rapid gas dispensal unit is used all component parts can be reused except for those that are sterilized by gamma rays (certain humidifier chambers). When steam autoclaves are used either in the ICU or in the station, these component must withstand temperatures of 120° to 136°C. Hytrel and silicone tubes are able to do this, but there are connectors which do not tolerate, these high temperatures. There are several cold liquid agents which are suitable as long as the manufacturer's instructions are strictly respected particularly as regards rinsing time. The advantage of this method is its simplicity.

Disinfection using a formal-ammoniac tight-housing apparatus can be used to sterilize a completely assembled ventilator, at the cost of a longer period of immobilization. The circuit parts must be perfectly dry. It is important that there are enough circuits and components available to equip the ventilator rapidly. There should be two complete circuits for each ventilator. If it is fitted with a removable expiratory block, one should allow one and a half to two blocks per ventilator according to the number in reserve (Chatburn 1989). Disposable sterile circuits matched to the different ventilators exist on the market. Their use simplifies the maintenance.

A disposable tubing circuit offers many advantages. Only the circuit components need sterilizing (du Cailar 1972) but the tubes are not always supplied sterile. The financial benefit must be evaluated. Due to their quality (resistance, transparency, and economy), polyethelyne tubes can be used to equip every ventilator; they are perfectly adapted to all simplified universal circuits for general use. The best are those which combine pliable and rigid sections and which resist stretching or compression, unlike nonstrengthened silicone tubing. In addition, this type of tubing is usually supplied in long rolls which can be divided as required. They can even be sterilized repeatedly in ethylene oxide gas!

Regular Circuit Replacement

When artificial ventilation first started, the method was to change the equipment after 1 week and send it away for cleaning, sterilizing, and checking. Since then ventilators have become much more reliable, and they can be used for longer periods provided the patient circuits are regularly replaced. Bacterial study of the water used in humidifiers has shown that it becomes contaminated after a few hours. It is therefore necessary not only to change the tubing of the circuit but also the humidifier. Ideally, this should be done daily, but every 2, 3 or 4 days is acceptable. If disposable parts are not used, there should be an adequate supply of components (Craven et al. 1988; Craven and Steger 1989; Lareau et al. 1978; Rieuf 1987; Simmons and Wang 1983; Tenaillon et al. 1988).

Bacterial filters with hydrophobic membranes are now available which remain permeable to gases saturated in water vapor for several days while retaining their antibacterial function. They are adapted to working in line with humidifiers equipped with a breathing tube heating system which keeps the ventilator gas at a temperature above condensation point (Bouilhac 1984). The answer is to use a bacterial filter placed in a suitable position:

1. In a universal simplified circuit (Fig. 1), the filter acts as an artificial nose which isolates the patient circuit (Chalon et al. 1984; Shelly et al. 1988; Tenaillon et al. 1989).
2. With the complete circuit (Fig. 2) instead of placing the filter at the humidifier outlet (Buckley 1984), it should be located at the extremity of the inspiratory

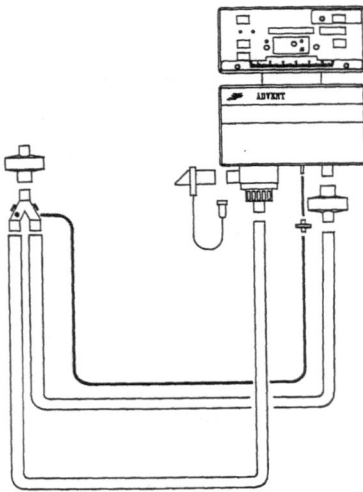

Fig. 1. A universal simplified circuit ventilator, with heat and moisture exchanger

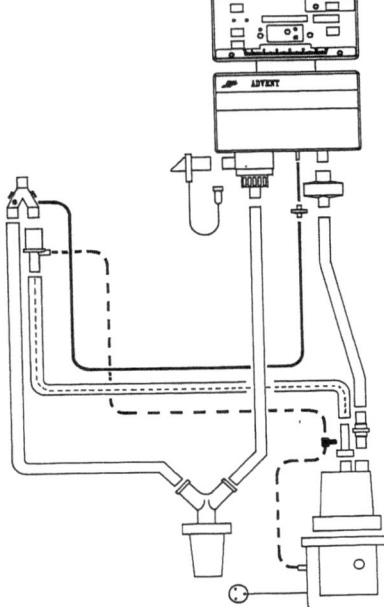

Fig. 2. Ventilator circuit fitted with a bacterial filter ventilator outlet

tube, connected to the Y-piece (Wolf 1984). This separates the circuit into two parts which then becomes a complete circuit with two bacterial, filters, having (a) in the first place an "inspiratory limb" from the ventilator outlet to the filter which is sterile, as long as the humidifier is filled from a bag; and (b) the "expiratory limb" with its water trap which also includes the filter, the Y-piece, and the patient adaptor; it has to be changed at suitable intervals. The filter can remain in use according to its performance (24, 48 h or longer according to the model), before being destroyed. Unfortunately, the ideal filter is not yet available; in fact if the membrane is of the hydrophobic type, it retains some humidity (as with the artificial nose), and this affects the working of the humidifier.

The first filter placed directly at the outlet of the ventilator isolates it from the patient circuit so that the ventilator is doubly protected from the ambient air and from the circuit itself. As only dry gas flows through it, it can remain in use for as long as 1000 h, provided one blocks off the outside outlet immediately after removing the circuit. When reassembling, the end piece should be thoroughly 2500 h (Rieuf 1987).

Daily Maintenance

Daily checks should be made of

—Heat and moisture exchanger with starting date
—Patient circuit and water traps

—Humidifier settings
—Nebulizer operating when used—drug nebulization may alter the accuracy of the expiratory flow transducers and generate some deposits within the expiratory valve
—Bacterial filter if mounted at end of inspiratory limb with date of installation, position, contamination; check above all that any malfunction of the humidifier does not turn the filter into an obstruction to expiratory flow (Buckley 1984);
—Condition of the ventilator and especially of the transducers (check the temperature of the heating elements, respirometer)
—Ventilator settings
—Alarm settings

These checks can be done with the routine checking of all the ventilators during daily physiotherapy. They must be recorded in the service checklist and patient record sheet whenever the ventilatory parameters are surveyed (Rieuf 1987). Because of his constant presence, the therapist best organizes the use of modular equipment, including the mounting of the circuits assembled in the unit (CPAP circuits), extra monitoring equipment and respiratory-therapy equipment (Incentive Respirometer, IPPB). Finally, he must keep up to date the ventilator and accessory records in which the problems and faults are entered, as well as the repair procedures with or without outside assistance.

Conclusion

This outline proposal is based on 15 years of experience. Other systems may be just as successful; however, we believe that constant attention to detail by the users on the spot is the best guarantee of success. Good maintenance, after all, is nothing else but constant attention to the multitude of details which added together make up the whole picture. Of course, the cost of this kind of operation is an important factor, especially if the intensive care unit is self-financing. On the other hand, a maintenance team of this type favors the introduction of the latest techniques and ventilators, thanks to its teaching support. It can equally participate in functional exploration at the bedside of the patient, as well as in the search for better circuits and the evaluation of new types of equipment.

References

Bouilhac M (1984) Filtre bactérien pour circuits de ventilation. Agressologie 25:299–302
Buckley PM (1984) Increase in resistance of in-line breathing filters humidified air. Br J Anaesth 56:637–643
Chalon J, Markham JP, Ali MM, Ramanathan S, Turndorf H (1984) The Pall Ultipor breathing circuit filter. An efficient heat and moisture exchanger. Anesth Analg 63:566–570

Chatburn RL (1989) Decontamination of respiratory care equipment. What can be done, what should be done. Respir Care 34:98–110

Craven DE, Steger KA (1989) Pathogenesis and prevention of nosocomial pneumonia in the mechanically ventilated patient. Respir Care 34:85–97

Craven DE, Connolly MG, Lichtenberg DA, Primeau PJ, McCabe WR (1982) Contamination of mechanical ventilators with tubing changes every 24 or 48 hours. N Engl J Med 306:1505–1509

Du Cailar J (1972) Utilisation du matériel à usage unique et des filtres bactériologiques en anesthésie et en réanimation respiratoire. Ann Anesthesiol Fr 13:427–428

Lareau SC, Ryan KJ, Diener CF (1978) The relationship between frequency of ventilator circuit changes and infetion hazard. Am Rev Respir Dis 118:493–496

Rieuf P (1987) La prévention de l'infection au cours de la ventilation artificielle. In: Ventilation artificielle conventionnelle et ventilation à haute fréquence. Arnette, Paris, pp 233–243

Shelly MP, Lloyd GM, Park GR (1988) A review of the mechanisms and methods of humidification of inspired gases. Intensive Care Med 14:1–9

Simmons BP, Wong ES (1983) Guideline for prevention of nosocomial pneumonia. Respir Care 28:221–232

Tenaillon A, Boiteau R, Froissard M, Normand F, Burdin M, Perrin-Gachadoat D (1988) Technologie et méthodologies de prévention des pneumopathies nosocomiales. In: Réanimation et Médecine d'Urgence. Expansion Scientifique Française, Paris, pp 262–268

Tenaillon A, Cholley G, Biteau R, Perrin-Gachadoat D, Burdin M (1987) Filtre échangeur de chaleur et d'humidité versus humidificateur chauffant en ventilation mécanique prolongée. Reanim Med Urgence 5:5–10

Wolf MA (1984) Elements d'hygiène de la ventilation artificielle. Agressologie 25:107–113

Appendix 1. Ohmeda Advent Preparation

1. Expiratory Module. Place the expiratory membrane inside the module with the spindle facing upwards. Position the module so that the horizontal "expiratory" outlet is on the right of the ventilator and secure it. The expiratory flow transducer must be connected to the horizontal expiratory outlet with the adaptor. Make sure that the transducer is the same as the one calibrated on the ventilator (each transducer has an identification number).
2. Humidifier. Fit the disposable chamber or the autoclavable one to the Fisher and Paykel heater base and secure it with the catch, lock.
3. Fit a refill bag full of sterile water on the tubing provided for this purpose. The 0.30-m tube attached to the connector of the refill circuit leads from the bacterial filter (A) to the humidifier chamber (inlet orifice).
4. Place the "patient circuit" in position.

—The inspiratory limb is composed of a 1.30-m tube, with a hose heater, attached to the temperature probe adaptor. It leads from the humidifier chamber outlet to the inspiratory branch of the Y-piece. When the bacterial filter (B) is used, it has to be located between the temperature probel adaptor and the Y-piece.

—The expiratory limb is composed of a 1.10-m tube, a water trap, and a 0.60-m tube. It leads from the expiratory branch of the Y-piece to the expiratory module inlet.

—The proximal airway pressure line leads from the ventilator outlet connector to the Y-piece connector (silicone tube, internal diameter = 6 mm) and operates with a bacteriological filter.
—The temperature probe is connected to the humidifier base, then to the hot wire adaptor (chamber outlet), and finally to the adaptor located on the Y-piece side of the inspiratory limb (this applies to Fisher and Paykel MR 500 and MR 600 humidifiers).

5. Finally, connect the heater element of the inspiratory limb to the power socket in the humidifier base.

Appendix 2. Preparation of Siemens Servo-Ventilator 900C

1. Expiratory channel (Fig. 3). Fit part *1* of the expiratory channel "expiration entry" to the front ventilatort socket. Place the safety water trap. Fit the silicone adaptors in sequence: cone-shaped *2, 4* onto the expiratory flow transducer *3* (after checking the fine net). Connect the electric plug linking the transducer to the ventilator electronics (check that the numbers are the same). Then fix the metal adaptor *5*, the silicone U piece, *6* (the arrow facing expiration), and the metal adaptor *7*. This part (7) must be connected to the electronic expiratory pressure transducer, inside the ventilator, with the tube plus bacterial filter (disposable), socket *10* (filter side). The expiratory pressure transducer is now connected to the expiratory channel. Insert the "expiratory outlet" **9** into the slot on the back panel of the ventilator. The rubber valve *8* links the adaptor *7* to part *9*. Check that it is not twisted. NB: Discard any rubber value which appears defective. Check that part no. 9 contains its nonreturn valve.
2. Humidifier. Fit the disposable chamber or the autoclavable one to the Fisher and Paykel heater base and secure it with the catch, lock.

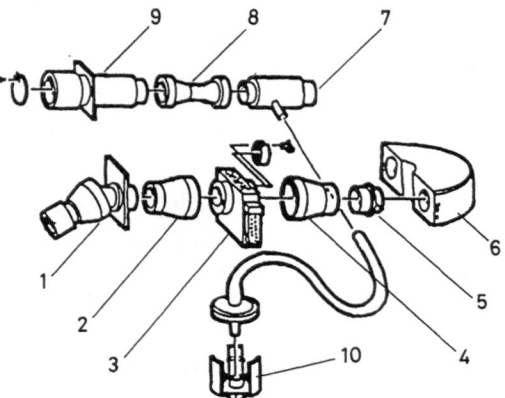

Fig. 3. Expiratory channel of Servo 900C

3. Fit a refill bag full of sterile water on the tubing provided for this purpose. The 0.30-m tube attched with the connector of the refill circuit leads from the bacterial filter (A) to the humidifier chamber (inlet orifice).

4. Place the "patient circuit" in position:

   —The inspiratory channel, with its hose heater, leads from the humidifier outlet to the temperature probe adaptor, which is itself fixed to the Y-piece.
   —The expiratory channel is composed of two 0.80-m tubes and a standard water trap. It leads from the Y-piece to the safety water trap of the ventilator.

5. The temperature probe connects to the base of the humidifier and then to the outlet adaptor of the humidifier chamber and finally to the adpator at the end of the Y-piece of the inspiratory channel (this applies to Fisher and Paykel MR 500 and MR 600 humidifiers).

6. Finally, connect the heating element of the inspiratory channel to the electrical input of the humidifier base.

Appendix 3. Advent Initial Adjustment

Mains switch "on/off" on back panel
$FiO_2 = 0.6$
Mode = Assist-controlled Ventilation
Frequency = 20 bpm
Tidal volume = 600 ml
Sensitivity = -2 hPa
Flow = 40 l
I:T = about 37%
Positive end expiratory pressure = 0
Pressure Support = 0
Inspiratory pause = 0.2 s
Ti = NA in assist-controlled
Sigh = off
Nebulizer = off
I:T limit = 50%
Apnea delay = 30 s
Maximum airway pressure = 60 hPa
Low airway pressure = 10 hPa
Low minute volume = 10 lpm
Low spontaneous Vt = off
High frequency = off
Humidifier heater (Fisher and Paykel) = on
Temperature setting = 36°C

Appendix 4. Initial adjustment of the Servo Ventilator 900C
(See Figs. 4, 5)

"On-Off" switch on back panel
$FiO_2 = 0.6$
Working pressure = 65 cm H_2O
Mode: controlled ventilation
Frequency = 20 breaths/min
Insufflation time = 25%; inspiratory pause = 10%
Minute Volume = 12 l/min
Flow form = See Appendix 3
Pressure Support = 0
SIMV frequency = 20 cycles/min (high rate)
Pressure alarm limit = 60 cm H_2O
Trigger = − 20 cm H_2O
"Adult" alarm limits
Low minute volume = 10 l/min
High volume/minute = 15 l/min
Positive expiratory pressure = 0
Tidal volume display
Low and high $FiO_2(0.5-0.7)$
Humidifier heater Fisher and Paykel = on
Temperature setting = 36°C

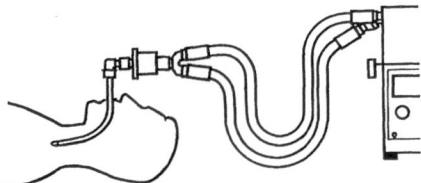

Fig. 4. Servo 900C with simplified universal circuit

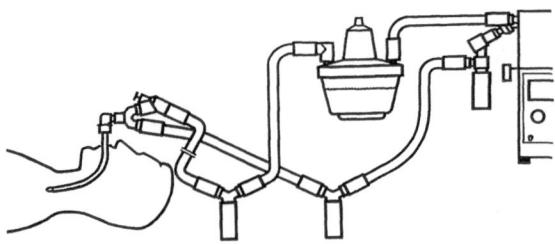

Fig. 5. Servo 900C with conventional patient circuit

Subject Index